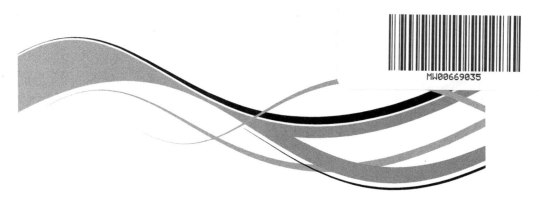

PHARMACY CERTIFIED
TECHNICIAN

Calculations
Workbook

EDITORS

Leah M. Ball, B.A.
Director of Communications
Michigan Pharmacists Association

Dianne E. Miller, R.Ph.
Chief Operations Officer
Michigan Pharmacists Association

FOURTH EDITION

Michigan Pharmacists Association
408 Kalamazoo Plaza, Lansing, MI 48933
MichiganPharmacists.org

The **PHARMACY CERTIFIED TECHNICIAN** Calculations Workbook
was developed by Michigan Pharmacists Association.

© 2015, 2010, 2003, 1994
Michigan Pharmacists Association
408 Kalamazoo Plaza, Lansing, MI 48933

CPhT™ is a federally registered trademark of the
Pharmacy Technician Certification Board (PTCB).
This book is in no way authorized by PTCB®.

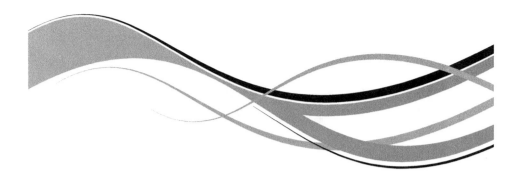

Table of Contents

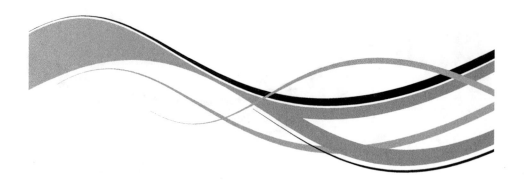

About the Authors

Leah Ball, B.A., is the director of communications with Michigan Pharmacists Association. She received her Bachelor of Arts degree in journalism, with concentrations in publication design and economics, from Michigan State University in East Lansing, Mich. At the Association, she oversees all publications, including the *Pharmacy Certified Technician Training Manual and Calculations Workbook,* *Michigan Pharmacist* journal, MichiganPharmacists.org, e-newsletters and social media, as well as advancing the pharmacy profession through public relations efforts and campaigns. She also recently served as the editor of *Michigan Pharmacy Law, Seventh Edition.*

Dianne E. Miller, R.Ph., received her Bachelor of Science degrees in pharmacy and applied biology in 1987 from Ferris State University in Big Rapids, Mich. She has completed a variety of certificate courses and post-graduate training, including the University of Pittsburgh's Smoking Cessation Specialist Certification Program, the National Institute for Pharmacists Outcomes Osteoporosis Care Certificate Program, University of Tennessee's Asthma Patient Management Certification Program and American Pharmacists Association's Pharmacy-Based Immunization Delivery Certificate Course. Miller is the Chief Operations Officer of Michigan Pharmacists Association in Lansing, Mich. She previously co-owned Miller's Pharmacy & Gift Shop, an independent community pharmacy in Grand Ledge, Mich. Prior to joining the staff at the Association, she was a staff pharmacist at Ingham Regional Medical Center in Lansing, Mich.

Karen Woods Miron, R.Ph., received her Bachelor of Science degree from Ferris State University (FSU) College of Pharmacy in Big Rapids, Mich., in 1974. Miron completed the Geriatric Consultant Pharmacist Certificate Program through FSU in 1994. Prior to retiring, Miron was the pharmacy manager for Walgreens OptionCare in Grand Rapids, Mich. She specialized in long-term care and home infusion for most of her career. She is a member of the American Society of Consultant Pharmacists, and previously served on the Executive Board of the Michigan Pharmacists Association. She currently serves on the Consultant Pharmacists Society of Michigan Board of Directors.

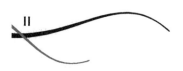

Theresa A. Mozug, CPhT, B.S., is the program director for the pharmacy technology programs at Henry Ford Community College in Dearborn, Mich. Over the span of more than 25 years at the college, Mozug has taught various courses within the program including calculations, pharmacology, computer software and pharmacy hands-on applications. Currently, she advises both pharmacy technicians and pre-pharmacy students in career planning, course selection and clinical rotations. She is the 2010 Michigan Society of Pharmacy Technicians (MSPT) Technician of the Year. Mozug earned a Bachelor of Science degree in health care services from the University of Phoenix.

Derek J. Quinn, Pharm.D., is the vice president of Westlake Drug in Kalamazoo, Mich. He received his Doctor of Pharmacy degree from Ferris State University in 2006 and has since received an immunization administration certificate and a diabetes medication therapy management certificate from the University of Findlay College of Pharmacy. Quinn is a preceptor for both student pharmacists and student pharmacy technicians. He previously served as an Executive Board member for Michigan Pharmacists Association.

Amal A. Sobh, Pharm.D., is a pharmacist with Garden City Hospital in Garden City, Mich. She received her Doctor of Pharmacy degree from Wayne State University Eugene Applebaum College of Pharmacy and Health Sciences, where she graduated with Rho Chi Honors. She serves as an adjunct faculty member at Henry Ford Community College for the Health Careers Division. Currently, she is teaching the pharmacy calculations course for the Pharmacy Technician Program. Sobh is also certified to deliver immunizations.

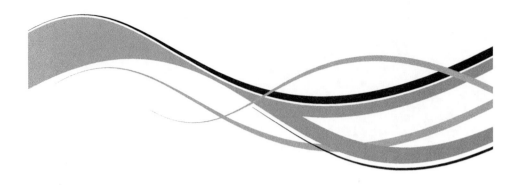

Acknowledgements

Michigan Pharmacists Association would like to thank Leah Ball and Nick Norcross, CPhT, for assistance in the editing process. MPA also acknowledges the following individuals for their contributions to the workbook: Linda Branoff, CPhT; Tabitha Cross; Jim Lile, Pharm.D.; Cathryn Poll, Pharm.D.; Derek Quinn, Pharm.D.; Michelle Richardson, CPhT; Cynthia Rowe; Stacy Ann Sipes; and La Vone Swanson.

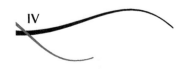

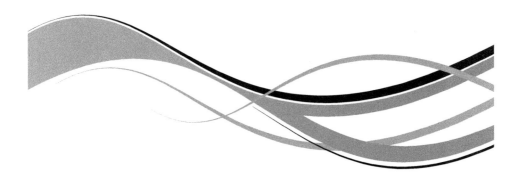

Introduction

The pharmacy technician has never been more critical to assisting the pharmacist's ever expanding role in cognitive services and patient care. Pharmacists depend on pharmacy technicians to accurately perform pharmacy calculations to support the medication distribution process.

This workbook has been developed to provide pharmacy technicians a foundation for commonly used pharmacy calculation functions. Not only does it review basic mathematic principles, but it brings pharmacy formulas and equations into real life situations that pharmacy technicians will encounter in practice.

How to Use This Workbook

Each chapter contains three basic elements: learning objectives, the main text with step-by-step examples and practice problems.

The learning objectives will give the reader a broad overview of the core concepts in each chapter. These are the elements that need to be mastered, so be sure to review before diving into the chapter, in order to measure understanding.

The main text of the chapters will provide key terms and definitions, memorization charts, formulas and equations to note, as well as real-life situations to which these calculations are applied. Each chapter includes working examples that take the learner step-by-step through the process.

At the end of each chapter, practice problems follow that reinforce key concepts and allow the learner to practically review.

This workbook comes with an accompanying CD-ROM, which includes answers to the practice problems, along with the work to solve each problem.

The Calculations Workbook is intended to be used in conjunction with the Pharmacy Certified Technician Training Manual, also produced by Michigan Pharmacists Association. Together, these materials should be helpful in preparing the pharmacy technician for the examination for national certification administered by the Pharmacy Technician Certification Board (PTCB), as well as providing a strong platform for technician career growth.

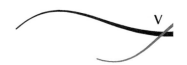

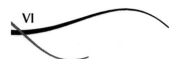

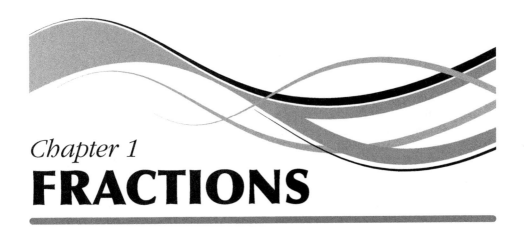

Chapter 1
FRACTIONS

By Theresa A. Mozug, CPhT, B.S.
Amal A. Sobh, Pharm.D.

Learning Objectives

Upon completion of this chapter, the technician should be able to:
- demonstrate a basic understanding of the "rules of fractions."
- convert fractions to lowest terms.
- convert improper fractions to mixed numbers and vice versa.
- perform fraction calculations involving addition, subtraction, multiplication and division.
- convert the verbal expression (written words) of a decimal number to its numerical value.
- learn the process of expressing decimal numbers as fractions.

Introduction

Though the concept of fractions is usually introduced to students in grade school, the application for pharmacy technicians can still be challenging if one doesn't remember the key concepts when adding, subtracting, multiplying and dividing fractions. Understanding the principles of fraction use is important as they are commonly used in dosages, measurements and other forms in practice. Reviewing the mathematical principles involving fractions will provide the pharmacy technician confidence in performing calculations involving algebra, proportions, dilutions and concentrations, among others.

Decimals are also regularly used in health care disciplines, including pharmacy. When pharmacy technicians have mastered the basic principles of the decimal system, they will have a strong foundation for working with measurement conversions, the metric system and medication dosages. Most prescriptions or medication orders include metric numbers, which rely on the decimal system. Studying mathematics involving fractions and decimals will increase the technician's accuracy and speed when dealing with these calculations.

Understanding Fractions

A fraction is a numerical representation that indicates a part or a division of some whole. Fractions appear as one number positioned above another number and separated by a line. They always consist of a **numerator** (the top number of the fraction) and a **denominator** (the bottom number of the fraction). This relationship of the part to the whole is shown in the fraction below.

2   numerator (the part)
—   fraction line
5   denominator (the whole)

The 5 (five) is the denominator (number below the bar), and it represents how many parts the whole is divided into or the sum of all the parts. The 2 (two) is the numerator (number above the bar) and represents the total number of parts. The fraction 2/5 can be expressed as two-fifths, two over five or two divided by five. A diagram to illustrate the concept of fractions can be seen in Figure 1.

Figure 1

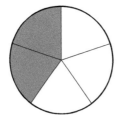

Proper or common fractions are fractions with a numerator less than the denominator (e.g., 3/10, 24/37, 9/564). The value of any proper or common fraction will be less than 1. **Mixed numbers** are fractions that include both a whole number and a proper fraction: 3 5/8, 15 6/11, 231 1/90. An **improper fraction** has a numerator equal to or larger than the denominator (e.g., 7/4, 53/11, 9/9). Improper fractions are equal to or greater than 1 and can be rewritten as mixed numbers. A **complex fraction** is a fraction in which the numerator and denominator are both fractions

(e.g., $\dfrac{\frac{1}{4}}{\frac{3}{8}}$, $\dfrac{\frac{5}{9}}{\frac{4}{5}}$).

General Principles of Fractions

There are two general principles to simplify mathematical calculations dealing with fractions.

Principle #1: For any fraction where both the numerator and denominator are multiplied or divided by the same number, the value of the fraction remains the same.

> **Tip:** Fractions that have the same value are called equivalent fractions. For example, 1/2 and 2/4 are equivalent fractions.

This principle is used when reducing fractions to lowest terms, as seen in the following example. Reducing fractions to lowest terms is sometimes called simplifying fractions. When working with a mixed number, set aside the whole number and simplify the fraction portion of the number. Once the fraction is reduced to its lowest term, place it beside the whole number.

EXAMPLE
Reducing a Fraction to Lowest Terms

Reduce 6/18 to lowest terms.

Step 1: Determine the largest whole number that can be divided into both the numerator and denominator.

List all the whole numbers that can be divided into 6 and 18.

The number 6 can be divided by the number 2 and 3.

The number 18 can be divided using the numbers 2, 3 or 6.

Step 2: Determine the largest whole number common to both the numerator and denominator and divide by that number.

The largest whole number common to both 6 and 18 is 6.

The numerator and denominator of the fraction 6/18 are then each divided by 6.

$$\frac{6}{18} \div \frac{6}{6} = \frac{1}{3}$$

Therefore, 6/18 reduced to lowest terms is 1/3.

Principle #2: The numerator should be smaller than the denominator. When the numerator is larger, the fraction is referred to as an "improper" fraction and must be reduced to a mixed number, which is a combination of a whole number and a fraction.

EXAMPLE

Converting an Improper Fraction to a Mixed Number

Convert 38/14 to a mixed number.

Step 1: First determine how many times the denominator can be divided into the numerator, which will become the whole number.

$$38 \div 14 = 2.71$$

The whole number in the mixed number becomes 2 since 38 can only be divided by 14 twice.

Step 2: To determine the fraction portion of the mixed number, multiply the denominator by the whole number determined in Step 1.

$$14 \times 2 = 28$$

Step 3: Subtract the answer to Step 2 from the original numerator, which becomes the new numerator that is placed over the original denominator.

$$38 - 28 = 10$$

The 10 becomes the new numerator and is placed over the original denominator. The resulting mixed fraction is 2 10/14.

Step 4: If possible, reduce the proper fraction for the final answer.

$$\frac{10}{14} \div \frac{2}{2} = \frac{5}{7}$$

Therefore, the correct answer and "proper" mixed fraction is 2 5/7.

Adding and Subtracting Fractions

Both adding and subtracting fractions require that the fractions have the same or common denominators. This process must occur before proceeding with any addition or subtraction calculation. In order to add or subtract fractions with different denominators, it is necessary to first find equivalent fractions with common denominators by finding the smallest multiple both denominators have in common. Then the fractions may be rewritten as equivalent fractions using a common denominator as the denominator for both fractions.

EXAMPLE
Adding Fractions

$$\frac{3}{5} + \frac{7}{9} =$$

Step 1: Find the equivalent fractions by multiplying each numerator and denominator by the other fraction's denominator.

$$\left(\frac{3}{5} \times \frac{9}{9}\right) + \left(\frac{7}{9} \times \frac{5}{5}\right) = \frac{27}{45} + \frac{35}{45}$$

Step 2: Add the numerators now that the fractions share a common denominator.

$$\frac{27 + 35}{45} = \frac{62}{45}$$

Step 3: If the addition results in an improper fraction, simplify to a mixed number. Be sure to reduce to lowest terms. (See example on page 3 for simplifying a mixed number.)

Therefore, the answer is 1 and 17/45.

EXAMPLE
Subtracting Fractions

$$\frac{3}{8} - \frac{1}{4} =$$

Step 1: Convert both denominators to create equivalent fractions.

In this example, both denominators can be evenly divided into the number 8, so only one of the fractions (1/4) must be converted to an equivalent fraction with a denominator of 8. This can be accomplished by simply multiplying 1/4 by 2/2.

$$\frac{1}{4} = \frac{(1 \times 2)}{(4 \times 2)} = \frac{2}{8}$$

The problem can now be rewritten as follows:

$$\frac{3}{8} - \frac{2}{8} =$$

Step 2: Subtract the numerators as the denominators are now equal.

$$\frac{(3-2)}{8} = \frac{1}{8}$$

Therefore, the final answer is 1/8.

Multiplying Fractions

Multiplying fractions is quite simple because it only requires multiplying numerators and denominators. When mixed numbers are involved in the calculations, they should be converted to improper fractions before being multiplied. Once the multiplication has been completed, the answer should be reduced to its lowest terms.

A technique called cancellation may be useful when multiplying fractions to reduce the size of the number being multiplied. This process saves time at the end of the problem because the resulting answer usually will be in lowest terms and will not require further reduction.

EXAMPLE
Multiplying Fractions

$$\frac{3}{7} \times \frac{7}{9} =$$

Step 1: Multiply the numerators and the denominators.

$$\frac{(3 \times 7)}{(7 \times 9)} = \frac{21}{63}$$

Step 2: Reduce the answer to lowest terms.

Both the numerator and the denominator are divisible by 21, so each can be divided by 21 in order to reduce the fraction.

$$\frac{21 \div 21}{63 \div 21} = \frac{1}{3}$$

OR

Step 1: Use the technique of cancellation.

Numbers may be able to be "cancelled" if they are the diagonally opposite numerator and denominator. With this problem, the 3 and 9 are diagonally opposite, as are the 7 and 7. If there is a number that can be divided into both, you can reduce the terms.

$$\frac{3}{7} \times \frac{7}{9} =$$

$$\frac{3 \div 3}{7} \times \frac{7}{9 \div 3} = \frac{1}{7} \times \frac{7}{3}$$

$$\frac{1}{7 \div 7} \times \frac{7 \div 7}{3} = \frac{1}{1} \times \frac{1}{3}$$

Step 2: After using cancellation, multiply the fraction.

$$\frac{1}{1} \times \frac{1}{3} = \frac{1}{3}$$

Therefore, the resulting answer is the same as using the multiplication method, 1/3.

EXAMPLE
Multiplying Mixed Fractions

$$7\frac{1}{4} \times 4\frac{5}{7} =$$

Step 1: Convert mixed fractions to improper fractions.

First, convert the mixed fraction 7 1/4 to an improper fraction by multiplying the whole number by the denominator then adding the numerator and placing the product over the denominator to obtain the equivalent fraction 29/4.

7 x 4 + 1 = 29; therefore, 7 1/4 = 29/4

4 x 7 + 5 = 33; therefore, 4 5/7 = 33/7

Step 2: Multiply the numerators and denominators of each improper fraction.

$$\frac{29}{4} \times \frac{33}{7} = \frac{(29 \times 33)}{(4 \times 7)} = \frac{957}{28}$$

Step 3: Convert improper fraction to mixed number of lowest terms. (See example on page 3 to convert improper fraction.)

Therefore, the final answer is 34 5/28.

Dividing Fractions

Dividing fractions involves some of the same steps as multiplying fractions, but one additional step is necessary. Dividing fractions is the same as multiplying one fraction by the reciprocal of another. To find the reciprocal, simply invert the **divisor** (number being divided by). Take note that the reciprocal of a whole number is one over that number. For example, the reciprocal of 1/5 is 5/1 or 5, and the reciprocal of 2 1/7 or 15/7 is 7/15.

When dividing, remember to convert mixed numbers to improper fractions before inverting the fraction on the right and multiplying the fractions. The final step is to reduce the answer to lowest terms.

EXAMPLE
Dividing Fractions

$$\frac{6}{8} \div \frac{1}{2} =$$

Step 1: Find the reciprocal of the divisor (invert the fraction).

$$\frac{1}{2} = \frac{2}{1}$$

Step 2: Multiply the fraction on the left by the reciprocal.

$$\frac{6}{8} \times \frac{2}{1} = \frac{(6 \times 2)}{(8 \times 1)} = \frac{12}{8}$$

Step 3: Convert the improper fraction to a mixed fraction and reduce to lowest terms.

$$\frac{12}{8} = 1\frac{4}{8} = 1\frac{1}{2}$$

Therefore, the answer is 1 1/2

EXAMPLE
Dividing Mixed Fractions

$$15\frac{1}{6} \div \frac{1}{3} =$$

Step 1: Convert the mixed fraction.

15 1/6 becomes the improper fraction 91/6.

The problem now becomes

$$\frac{91}{6} \div \frac{1}{3} =$$

Step 2: Multiply by the reciprocal of the fraction on the right.

$$\frac{91}{6} \times \frac{3}{1} = \frac{(91 \times 3)}{(6 \times 1)} = \frac{273}{6}$$

Step 3: Convert the improper fraction to a mixed number and simplify the resulting fraction.

$$\frac{273}{6} = 45\frac{3}{6} = 45\frac{1}{2}$$

Therefore, the final answer is 45 and 1/2.

Decimals

Whole numbers include numbers like 0, 1, 2 and 3, but not every number is a whole number. The **decimal system** is a method used to express and write numbers that are fractions, as well as whole numbers, using a symbol called the **decimal point**. The decimal point represents the boundary between a whole number and a portion of a number or fraction. Any number to the left of the decimal point is a **whole number** and any number to the right of the decimal point is a **decimal number**. Decimals are actually fractions with a denominator of any multiple of 10 (e.g., 10, 100, 1,000, 10,000) determined by the number's position following the decimal point. When there is no whole number present, a decimal number's value is always less than 1.

> **Tip:** Health care professionals often place a zero to the left of the decimal point for any decimal that does not include a whole number to emphasize that the number is less than 1. In this way, many errors have been eliminated that may have been caused by misreading a decimal number, especially when interpreting dosages.

Reading Decimal Numbers

In the decimal number system, the value of a digit depends on its place or location in the number. Each place has a value of 10 times the place to its right. As you move right from the decimal point, each place value is divided by 10. To read decimal numbers, say the numbers to the right as if they were whole numbers, then add the decimal place value. For example, the decimal number 325.263 is read as "three hundred twenty-five and two hundred sixty-three thousandths." (See Figure 2.) The "th" at the end of a word means less than one or a fraction part, indicating the number is to the right of the decimal point. (Although less common, the number could also be read as "three hundred twenty-five point two six three.")

Figure 2

thousands	hundreds	tens	ones	and	tenths	hundredths	thousandths	ten thousandths	hundred thousandths
	3	2	5	.	2	6	3		
	Whole Numbers				Numbers less then 1				

EXAMPLE
Writing Decimal Numbers That Are Less Than One

Write the number one hundred eighty-five thousandths in a decimal form.

> The "th" on thousandths indicates the number is less than one.

> Therefore, the number is written as 0.185.

EXAMPLE
Writing Decimals Numbers That Are Greater Than One

Write the number four hundred thirty-five and two tenths in decimal form.

> The "and" separates the whole number from the decimal number, just as the decimal point does when written in numerical form. The "th" indicates the decimal portion that is less than one.

> Therefore, the number is written as 435.2.

Converting Fractions to Decimals

To convert a fraction to a decimal, simply divide the numerator by the denominator. This can be a useful method for determining whether two fractions are equal. If the resulting decimal numbers are the same, then the fractions are equal.

EXAMPLE
Converting a Fraction to a Decimal

$$\frac{1}{6} =$$

> Divide the numerator by the denominator.

> $1 \div 6 = 0.16$

Therefore, the decimal equivalent of 1/6 is 0.16

Converting Decimals to Fractions

To convert a decimal to a fraction, use the decimal number as a whole number to express the numerator of the fraction. The denominator becomes the decimal place value, and the fraction is reduced to lowest terms.

EXAMPLE
Converting a Decimal to a Fraction

Convert the number 0.234 to a fraction.

Step 1: Convert to a fraction.

The decimal can be read as two hundred and thirty-four thousandths. Therefore, the denominator is 1,000 and the numerator is 234.

$$\frac{234}{1,000}$$

Step 2: Reduce the fraction to lowest terms by dividing the numerator and the denominator by the largest number that both numbers can be divided into evenly.

$$\frac{234 \div 2}{1,000 \div 2} = \frac{117}{500}$$

Therefore, 0.234 is equal to the fraction $\frac{117}{500}$.

Rounding Decimals

Decimals are often rounded in health care to create manageable numbers. Working with a number that has multiple digits, such as 64.195638, can result in calculation errors due to the number of digits involved and the complexity of adding, subtracting, multiplying or dividing a decimal number with so many digits. It is much easier to work with the number 64.2. Rounding to a specific decimal place is accomplished in the same way that whole numbers are rounded. It is generally acceptable to round decimal numbers to the nearest tenth or the nearest hundredth. When rounding to the tenth or hundredth digit, evaluate the number following that digit on the right. If that number is 5 or greater, add 1 to the preceding digit and drop all the numbers to the right of the changed number. If that number is less than 5, leave the preceding digit the same and drop all the numbers to the right of that number that was left unchanged.

EXAMPLE
Rounding Decimal Numbers

Round 2.86 to the nearest tenth.

The tenth digit in 2.86 is held by the number 8.

The number to the right of the 8 is 6, so 1 should be added to the number 8 to equal 9. All the numbers to the right of the tenth digit are dropped, as seen below.

2.86 = 2.9

Significant Figures

A **significant decimal place or figure** is one that is actually measured. The number of significant digits reported is dependent upon the accuracy of the measuring device used or the decimal places in each of the numbers used in a calculation (see example on determining significant figures in a calculation on the next page). When a mathematical problem (adding, subtracting, multiplying or dividing) involves decimal numbers with differing significant figures, the answer should be reported with the least number of decimal places in any one number.

The rules for assigning significant figures are as follows:

1. Figures other than zero are always significant.
    For example, 56.15 has four significant figures.

2. Leading zeros to the left of the first nonzero digit are never significant.
    For example, 0.008 has one significant figure.

3. Trailing zeros after a decimal point may or may not be significant depending on the problem. For example, 0.0080 may have two significant figures: the eight and the last zero or only one significant figure, just the 8, depending on the problem.

4. Zeros between two other significant digits are always significant.
    For example, 50.3 has three significant digits.

EXAMPLE
Determining Significant Figures

Determine the number of significant figures in 3.6203.

> Since zeros between two other significant digits are always significant, the number of significant figures in 3.6203 is 5.

EXAMPLE
Determining Significant Figures in a Calculation

$4.68562 \times 1.52 =$

> The product is 7.1221424. However, the answer must be rounded to the hundredths place because the answer can only be reported to the least accurate space value. Since 1.52 was only accurate to the hundredths place, the answer can only be accurate to the hundredths place. Therefore, the answer can be reported as 7.12.

EXAMPLE
Determining Significant Figures in a Calculation

$3.89752 \times 4.345 =$

> The product is 16.9347244. However, the answer must be rounded to the thousandths place because the answer can only be reported to the least accurate space value. Since 4.345 was only accurate to the thousandths place, the answer can only be accurate to the thousandths place. Therefore, the answer can be reported as 16.935.

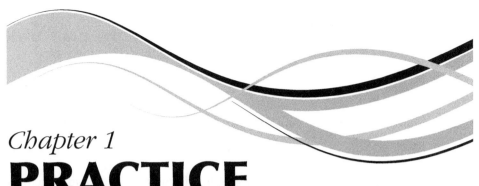

Chapter 1
PRACTICE PROBLEMS

Reduce the following fractions to lowest terms.

1. 6/18
2. 8/48
3. 9/24
4. 21/294
5. 42/144

Convert the improper fractions to mixed numbers.

6. 84/22
7. 6/5
8. 33/12
9. 186/61
10. 87/9

Convert the mixed numbers to improper fractions.

11. 3 8/13
12. 2 4/71
13. 2 1/4
14. 2 7/8
15. 1 53/54

Perform the mathematical calculations specified to add and subtract fractions. Reduce to lowest terms and/or convert to a mixed number when necessary.

16. 3/21 + 8/7

17. 5/8 + 1/6

18. 36/45 – 5/9

19. 7/4 – 6/12

Perform the mathematical calculations specified to multiply and divide fractions. Reduce to lowest terms and/or convert to a mixed number when necessary.

20. 3/7 x 1 2/3

21. 3/8 x 9/10

22. 13/15 x 2 1/2

23. 4/5 x 11/12

24. 9 3/8 x 3/4

25. 1/3 ÷ 5/6

26. 4 8/9 ÷ 2 3/7

27. 7 ÷ 1 3/5

28. 1/2 ÷ 4/5

29. 19/22 ÷ 3

Convert the written expressions for decimals into numbers.

30. Three hundred two and sixty-nine thousandths

31. Twenty-four and eight-tenths

32. Six thousand six hundred seventy-one and fifteen hundredths

33. Two hundred seventy-five thousandths

34. Nine-hundredths

Convert the fractions to decimal numbers.

35. 2/5

36. 7/18

37. 42/75

38. 7/4

39. 65/260

40. 126/360

41. 1,462/11,696

42. 22/8

Convert the decimal numbers to fractions or mixed numbers in lowest terms.

43. 0.45

44. 155.2

45. 0.475

46. 29.002

Round the decimal numbers as directed.

47. 23.282 to the nearest tenth

48. 16,730.54918 to the nearest thousandth

Determine the number of significant figures.

49. 0.00935

50. 345.1072

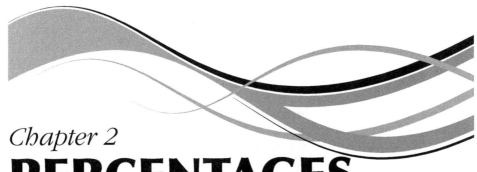

Chapter 2
PERCENTAGES, RATIOS AND PROPORTIONS

By   Theresa A. Mozug, CPhT, B.S.
     Amal A. Sobh, Pharm.D.

Learning Objectives

Upon completion of this chapter, the technician should be able to:
■   define the concept of percent and percentages.
■   convert fractions and decimal numbers to percents.
■   convert percentages to fractions and decimals.
■   define ratios and proportions.
■   convert ratios to decimals, fractions and percentages.
■   learn how to solve for an unknown value using a proportion.

Introduction

Pharmacy professionals must have a solid working knowledge of percents so they can perform important everyday pharmacy services calculations, such as percent strength of solutions for patient medications, preparing intravenous solutions or dispensing ointments labeled with percents. Technicians continue to play an increasingly involved role in dispensing functions and the compounding process, requiring appropriate skills to execute percent calculations.

Applications of ratios and proportions are implemented daily in a busy pharmacy, and up to three-quarters of the calculations the pharmacy technician will perform involves these concepts. Competency is essential, because dosage calculations based on age and/or weight are critical for all patients, especially infants, cancer patients and the elderly.

Understanding Percentages

The term **percent** and its corresponding symbol (%) means "by the hundred" or "in a hundred," and **percentage** means "parts per hundred." Percents are an example of a part to whole relationship in math. Percent is basically a reference to the numerator in a fraction with a denominator of 100. Percents may also be expressed as a ratio or represented as a common or decimal fraction. For example, 49% means 49 parts in 100 and may be expressed as a ratio, 49:100; a fraction, 49/100; or a decimal, 0.49.

The following equation represents the concept of percentages and can be used to interpret the numerical value of a percent.

$$\frac{\%}{100} = \frac{\text{number of parts}}{\text{total number of parts of the whole}}$$

EXAMPLE
Determining the Numerical Value of a Percent

What is the value of 68%?

If percent is defined as parts per hundred, 68% can indicate any of the following:

- 68 parts per 100
- 68:100 as a ratio
- 68/100 as a fraction
- 0.68 as a decimal

Tip: Remember that percent means "parts per hundred."

Conversions Between Percents, Fractions and Decimals

Converting fractions and decimals to percents and vice versa is a simple mathematical process involving multiplication and division.

To convert a fraction or decimal number into a percentage:
1. Divide the numerator by the denominator to get a decimal number.
2. Convert the decimal to the percent by multiplying the decimal number by 100 and adding the % sign.

3. OR, use the simplified multiplication method. This easier method of converting a decimal to a percent can be accomplished by shifting the decimal point two places to the right. Remember to always use the decimal point as the starting point for a percent conversion and that it is possible to have percentages greater than 100.

EXAMPLE
Converting Fractions to Percents

Convert $\frac{3}{6}$ to a percent.

Step 1: Divide the numerator by the denominator to get a decimal.

$3 \div 6 = 0.50$

Step 2: Convert the decimal to a percent by multiplying the decimal number by 100, and add the percent sign to the resulting number.

$0.50 \times 100 = 50$

Therefore, $\frac{3}{6} = 50\%$

OR, you can also use the simplified multiplication method by shifting the decimal point two places to the right. Then add the % sign to the number.

$.50 = 50$
‿‿
1 2

Therefore, the final answer is 50%.

EXAMPLE
Converting Percentages to Decimals

Convert 76% to a decimal.

This problem can be solved in two different manners. First, percent can be converted to a decimal by dividing the percent number by 100.

$76\% = 76 \div 100 = 0.76$

Therefore, 76% can be expressed as the decimal 0.76.

You can also solve the problem using simplified division by moving the decimal point two places to the left.

$$76\% = 76.0 = .76$$
$$\underset{2\ \ 1}{\smile\smile}$$

Therefore, the final answer is 0.76, regardless of which method is used.

To convert a percentage to a decimal or fraction:
- Divide the percent number by 100.
- OR, shift the decimal point two places to the left. This process of quick division replaces having to divide the number by 100 and is the method known as simplified division.
- Convert the percentage to a fraction by removing the % sign, placing that number over 100 and reducing to lowest terms.

EXAMPLE
Converting Percentages to Fractions

Convert 12.5% to a fraction.

Step 1: Divide percent number by 100, as percent is defined as parts per hundred.

12.5% can be converted to a fraction using 12.5 as the numerator and 100 as the denominator.

$$\frac{12.5}{100}$$

Step 2: Simplify the fraction to lowest terms.

$$\frac{12.5 \div 12.5}{100 \div 12.5} = \frac{1}{8}$$

Therefore, 12.5% is equivalent to the fraction 1/8.

Solving Percentage Problems

Percent problems can be solved using the equation illustrated earlier in the chapter or using a method called proportions, which will be explained later in this chapter. Using the following formula, one can solve any percent problem when three of the values are known. The known values are inserted into the formula and the unknown value is determined. It is important to insert the known value in the correct place in the formula to ensure the answer is correct.

$$\frac{\%}{100} = \frac{\text{number of parts}}{\text{total number of parts of the whole}}$$

This equation can also be expressed as follows:
% needed x total number of parts of the whole =
number of parts for the % needed

EXAMPLE
Solving Percentage Problems

What is 40% of 75?

Step 1: Using the formula, insert the known values.

$$\frac{\%}{100} = \frac{\text{number of parts}}{\text{total number of parts of the whole}}$$

$$\frac{40}{100} = \frac{Z}{75}$$

Step 2: Solve for the missing value.

Multiply both sides by 75 to isolate Z.

$$\frac{75}{1} \times \frac{40}{100} = \frac{Z}{75} \times \frac{75}{1}$$

$$\frac{75 \times 40}{100} = Z$$

$$\frac{3,000}{100} = Z$$

OR, cross multiply diagonally to solve for the unknown (Z).

(100 x Z) = (40 x 75)

100Z = 3,000

Divide each side of the equation by 100.

$$\frac{\cancel{100}\,Z}{\cancel{100}} = \frac{3,000}{100}$$

Step 3: Simplify the fraction to a whole number.

$$Z = \frac{3,000}{100} = 30$$

Therefore, 40% of 75 is the number 30.

You can also solve the problem using the alternative equation:
% needed x total number of parts of the whole = number of parts for the % needed

Step 1: Insert the known values into the equation.

40% x 75 = Z

Step 2: Solve for the unknown by converting the percent to a decimal and multiplying.

0.40 x 75 = Z

30 = Z

Therefore, the answer is 30, regardless of the formula used.

Tip: The word "of" means to multiply. For example, if solving for 40% of 100, simply multiply 40% by 100.

EXAMPLE
Solving Percentage Problems

What percent of 200 is 12?

Step 1: Insert the known values into the equation.

$$\frac{X\%}{100} = \frac{12}{200}$$

Step 2: Solve for the missing value.

Multiply both sides by 100 to isolate X.

$$\frac{\cancel{100}}{1} \times \frac{X\%}{\cancel{100}} = \frac{12}{200} \times \frac{100}{1}$$

$$X\% = \frac{1,200}{200}$$

OR, cross multiply diagonally to solve for the unknown (X).

$(X\% \times 200) = (100 \times 12)$

$200X\% = 1,200$

Divide each side by 200.

$$\frac{\cancel{200}X\%}{\cancel{200}} = \frac{1,200}{200}$$

Step 3: Reduce to lowest terms.

$$X\% = \frac{1,2\cancel{00}}{2\cancel{00}} = 6$$

Therefore, 12 is 6% of 200.

Percents sometimes include fractions, which complicates calculations involving them. The best way to manage these percents is to treat them as complex fractions. It is not advisable to change the fraction to a decimal, because the answer may not be as exact when compared to the fraction calculation. The problem should be set up in a proportion format to solve for the answer.

EXAMPLE
Solving Percentage Problems
Involving Fractions

What is 12 1/4% of 275?

Step 1: Insert the known values into the equation.

$$\frac{12\frac{1}{4}\%}{100} = \frac{Z}{275}$$

Step 2: Convert the percent to an complex fraction.

12 1/4% converted to an complex fraction is 49/4.

$$\frac{\frac{49}{4}}{100} = \frac{Z}{275}$$

Step 3: Cross multiply diagonally to solve for the unknown (Z).

$$(100 \times Z) = (49/4 \times 275)$$

$$100Z = \frac{49}{4} \times \frac{275}{1}$$

$$100Z = \frac{13,475}{4}$$

$$4 \times 100Z = \frac{13,475}{4} \times 4$$

$$400Z = 13,475$$

$$\frac{400Z}{400} = \frac{13,475}{400}$$

$$Z = 33.6875$$

Therefore, 12 1/4% of 275 is 33.6875 or 33.7.

Tip: When dividing fractions, the divisor should be converted to a reciprocal fraction and then multiplied.

EXAMPLE
Solving Percentage Problems Involving Fractions

What is 5 1/4% of 130?

Step 1: Insert the known values into the formula.
% needed x total number of parts of the whole = number of parts for the % needed

$$5\frac{1}{4}\% \times 130 = X$$

Step 2: Convert the percent to an improper fraction.

$$\frac{21}{4}\% \times 130 = X$$

Step 3: Convert the percent to an improper fraction and solve for the unknown (X).

$$\left(\frac{21}{4} \times \frac{1}{100}\right) \times 130 = X$$

$$\frac{21}{400} \times \frac{130}{1} = X$$

$$X = \frac{2{,}730}{400} = 6.825$$

Step 4: Convert the improper fraction to a mixed number and reduce to lowest terms.

$$6 \times 400 = 2{,}400 \quad 2{,}730 - 2{,}400 = 330$$

$$X = 6\frac{330}{400} = 6\frac{33}{40}$$

Therefore, 5 1/4% of 130 is 6 33/40.

EXAMPLE
Solving Percentage Problems Involving Decimals

What percent of 120 is 55.2?

Step 1: Insert the known values into the equation.

$$\frac{X\%}{100} = \frac{55.2}{120}$$

Step 2: Solve for the missing value.

Multiply both sides by 100 to isolate X.

$$\frac{100}{1} \times \frac{X\%}{100} = \frac{55.2}{120} \times \frac{100}{1}$$

$$X\% = \frac{552}{12}$$

$$X\% = 46$$

OR, cross multiply diagonally to solve for the unknown (X).

$$(X\% \times 120) = (100 \times 55.2)$$

$$120X\% = 5,520$$

$$\frac{\cancel{120}\,X\%}{\cancel{120}} = \frac{5,520}{120}$$

$$X\% = 46$$

Therefore, 55.2 is 46% of 120.

Ratios

A **ratio** is used to express a relationship between two numbers. These numbers are usually separated by a colon (:), as in 7:2. The colon that separates the two numbers is expressed as "is to." Therefore, the above example would be verbally expressed as "7 is to 2." Two sets of numbers can be compared to each other using two colons. An example is 3:6::6:12. This example can be expressed verbally as "3 is to 6 as 6 is to 12," where the "::" means "=".

The numbers in a ratio refer to parts of one substance as compared to parts of another substance. The ratio 4:5 might refer to four parts of simple syrup to five parts of wild cherry syrup. The units of measurement associated with the "parts" could be weight, volume or even objects like grapefruits or tablets. When comparing ratios, it is important to remember that the units must be the same; the units in the numerators must match and the units in the denominators must match.

Several types of conversions can be performed using ratios. One frequently used conversion involves changing a ratio to a fraction or vice versa. A ratio can easily be converted to a fraction by replacing the colon with a slanted line (fraction bar), then reducing the newly created fraction to lowest terms. To convert a fraction to a ratio, simply reverse the process by reducing the fraction to lowest terms and replace the slanted line (fraction bar) with a colon.

EXAMPLE
Converting a Ratio to a Fraction

Convert 2:8 to a fraction.

$$2:8 = \frac{2}{8} = \frac{1}{4}$$

Therefore, the ratio 2:8 is equal to the fraction 1/4.

Converting a ratio into a decimal is also a simple process. First convert the ratio into a fraction, then divide the numerator by the denominator. The resulting decimal can also be converted to a percent, if necessary, by multiplying the decimal by 100 and adding the % sign. Likewise, a percent can be converted to a ratio by removing the % sign, placing that number over 100, reducing the fraction to lowest terms and replacing the slanted line (fraction bar) with a colon.

EXAMPLE
Converting a Fraction to a Ratio

Convert 8/16 to a ratio.

Step 1: Reduce fraction to lowest terms.

$$\frac{8}{16} = \frac{1}{2}$$

Step 2: Convert to a ratio.

$$\frac{1}{2} = 1:2$$

Therefore, 8/16 is equal to the ratio 1:2.

EXAMPLE
Converting a Ratio to a Percent

Convert 1:4 to a percent.

Step 1: Convert the ratio to a fraction.

$$1:4 = \frac{1}{4}$$

Step 2: Convert the fraction to a decimal.

$$1 \div 4 = 0.25$$

Step 3: Convert the decimal to a percent.

Multiply the decimal by 100, and add the % sign.
$0.25 \times 100 = 25\%$

Therefore, the ratio 1:4 is equal to 25%.

EXAMPLE
Converting a Percent to a Ratio

Convert 30% to a ratio.

Step 1: Convert the percent to a fraction and reduce to lowest terms.

$$30\% = \frac{30}{100} = \frac{3}{10}$$

Step 2: Convert the fraction to a ratio.

$$\frac{3}{10} = 3:10$$

Therefore, 30% is equal to the ratio 3:10.

Proportions

A proportion compares two ratios to one another. Proportions can be used in a wide variety of health care applications. They also provide a simple method of solving many everyday math problems, such as cooking measurement conversions, increasing or decreasing ingredient amounts or mixing cleaning substances. For example, 4/6 equals 8/12 or 4:6::8:12.

Proportion concepts allow the pharmacy technician to solve for an unknown (Y) when the other three values are known. To solve for the unknown (Y), cross multiplication is used. To do this, set up the problems as fractions. When beginning a problem, place the like measurements [such as milligrams and milligrams (mg), and milliliters and milliliters (mL)] across from each other.

EXAMPLE
Using a Proportion to Solve For an Unknown (Y)

(Note: In this problem, when comparing two ratios, the units in the numerators are the same and the units in the denominators are the same.)

6 mg : 2 mL :: Y mg : 30 mL

Step 1: Convert proportion to a fraction equation.

$$\frac{6 \text{ mg}}{2 \text{ mL}} = \frac{Y \text{ mg}}{30 \text{ mL}}$$

Step 2: Cross multiply to solve for the unknown (Y).

Y mg x 2 = 6 x 30

2Y mg = 180

$$\frac{2Y \text{ mg}}{2} = \frac{180}{2}$$

Y = 90 mg

Therefore, 6 mg is to 2 mL as 90 mg is to 30 mL.

EXAMPLE
Using a Proportion to Solve a Practical Problem For an Unknown

A patient weighs 150 pounds. The doctor ordered a drug that has a dosage dependent on milligrams (mg) of medication per kilogram of body weight. The pharmacy technician will need to convert pounds to kilograms, using the ratio of 1 kg : 2.2 pounds.

Step 1: Convert the ratio to a fraction equation.

$$\frac{1 \text{ kg}}{2.2 \text{ lbs}} = \frac{Y \text{ kg}}{150 \text{ lbs}}$$

Step 2: Cross multiply to solve for the unknown (X).

Y kg x 2.2 = 150 x 1

2.2Y kg = 150

$$\frac{2.2Y}{2.2} = \frac{150}{2.2}$$

Y = 68.18 kg

Therefore, 150 pounds is equivalent to 68.18 kg.

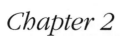

Chapter 2

PRACTICE PROBLEMS

Convert the following decimals to percents.

1. 0.47

2. 1.69

3. 3.8

4. 0.0025

Convert the following percents to decimals.

5. 135%

6. 33%

7. 0.4%

8. 19%

Convert the following fractions to percents.

9. 11/22

10. 1 7/8

11. 1/4

12. 6/10

Convert the following percents to fractions.

13. 98%

14. 55%

15. 15 1/5%

16. 20%

Solve the following practical problems involving percentages.

17. What is 60% of 75?

18. What is 8 1/4% of 200?

19. What percentage of 250 is 46?

20. What percent of 54 is 189?

Convert the following ratios to fractions.

21. 6:15

22. 4:20

23. 15:45

24. 21:49

Convert the following fractions to ratios.

25. 3/5

26. 13/15

27. 1/9

28. 7/8

Convert the following ratios to percents.

29. 6:8

30. 4:10

31. 2:5

32. 5:20

Convert the following percents to ratios.

33. 33%

34. 46%

35. 65%

36. 8%

Solve for the unknown in the following proportions.

37. 4.5:9 :: X:50

38. X:12 :: 3:4

39. 1:X :: 5:12

40. 5:8 :: 22:X

Solve the following practical problems involving proportions.

41. A pediatric patient is ordered a dose of 2.5 mL of amoxicillin. If amoxicillin is available as a 125 mg/5 mL suspension, how many mg is the patient receiving?

42. If clindamycin injection is available as a 900 mg/6 mL vial, how many mL are needed to fill a clindamycin 300 mg order?

43. Vancomycin is compounded as a 1,000 mg/40 mL oral suspension. If a patient's dose is 250 mg, how many mL will be administered?

44. If an IV solution is labeled as 0.45% sodium chloride, how many grams of sodium chloride will a 1 L bag contain?

45. If a 50 mL syringe contains 12.5 g of dextrose, what percent of dextrose does the syringe contain? (Note: % = X g/100 mL)

46. If a patient weighs 264 lbs, how much does the patient weigh in kg? (Note: 2.2 lbs = 1 kg)

47. If a patient weighs 88 kg, how much does the patient weigh in lbs?

48. Acetaminophen extra strength tablets are available as 500 mg tablets. If a patient was prescribed a dose of 1,000 mg of extra strength acetaminophen, how many tablets will he need to take?

49. A patient presents with a compound of 20 g of hydrocortisone combined with 10 g of zinc oxide. What is the ratio of hydrocortisone to the total amount of the compound?

50. Using the information in the previous problem, what percentage of the compound is zinc oxide?

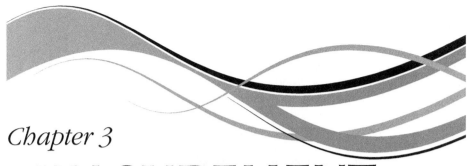

Chapter 3

MEASUREMENT SYSTEMS

By   Dianne E. Miller, R.Ph.
Jill Cobb, B.A.

Learning Objectives

Upon completion of this chapter, the technician should be able to:
- identify the three basic units of measure used in the metric system.
- explain the meanings of the prefixes most commonly used in metric measurements.
- convert metric measurements to express different metric units.
- understand the differences and similarities between the apothecary and avoirdupois systems of measurement.
- convert apothecary measurements to express different apothecary units.
- convert avoirdupois measurements to express different avoirdupois units.
- describe how household measurements are used in pharmacy practice.
- convert apothecary measurements to equivalent metric measurements.
- convert avoirdupois measurements to equivalent metric measurements.

Introduction

The metric system is the most commonly and frequently used system of measure in pharmacy practice. However, other systems, including the apothecary, avoirdupois and household systems of measurement, occasionally appear in pharmacy and medical systems. Pharmacy technicians must be familiar with each system and how to convert between each system as a basic function of procedure.

The Metric System

The **metric system** is a logical decimal system based on multiples of 10 (0.001, 0.01, 0.1, 1, 10, 100, 1,000 and so on). For this reason, metric numbers are expressed as whole numbers or decimal numbers, but never as fractions. Metric notations also have a direct correlation between units of measure, such as length, volume and weight, making mathematical calculations quite simple once basic principles are understood.

Decimals and metric measurements are based on units of 10. There are three basic units of measure in the metric system.

- Meter (m) = unit of length
- Gram (g) = unit of weight
- Liter (L) = unit of volume

To specify a particular measure, one can add prefixes (syllables placed at the beginning of words) to these basic units. Each prefix denotes powers of 10, as illustrated in Table 1.

Table 1

Common Metric Prefixes and Meanings

Prefix	Meaning	Value	Symbol
kilo-	one thousand (basic unit 10^3 or unit x 1,000)	1,000	k
hecto-	one hundred (basic unit x 10^2 or unit x 100)	100	h
deka-	ten (basic unit x 10^1 or unit x 10)	10	da
base	one	1	m, g, L
deci-	one tenth or 1/10 (basic unit x 10^{-1} or unit x 0.1)	0.1	d
centi-	one hundredth or 1/100 (basic unit x 10^{-2} or unit x 0.01)	0.01	c
milli-	one thousandth or 1/1,000 (basic unit x 10^{-3} or unit x 0.001)	0.001	m
micro-	one millionth 1/1,000,000 (basic unit x 10^{-6} or unit x 0.000001)	0.000001	mc or μ

Every metric prefix may be combined with every basic unit or root. The application of these terms depends on the measurement being completed. Thus, liquids are measured as units of volume in liters and dry medications use grams as a measure of weight. Table 1 demonstrates commonly used prefixes with each of the basic units of measure.

Metric conversion problems can be easily solved by moving the decimal either to the left (to convert from smaller units to larger units) or the right (to convert from larger units to smaller units).

Use of a mnemonic device may be helpful to keep the metric units in the correct sequence or order. Try something silly like "**K**ind **h**elpful **d**aughters **b**ring **d**elicious **c**hocolate **mi**nts, **Mo**m." The first letter of each word in the silly sentence represents the first letter of the units. The "mi" in mints should help one distinguish milli-, which ends with an "i," comes before micro-, which ends with an "o," and is represented by the "mo" in mom. Knowing a technique like this will help you remember the order of the units on an exam.

Conversions Within the Metric System

To change units within the metric system, review the number's place value and consider the place value of the desired unit. Count the number of spaces from the beginning number to the ending unit.

Table 2
Common Metric Units

Length: Basic unit = meter 1 millimeter (mm) = 1/1,000 of a meter = 1,000 micrometers (µm) 1 centimeter (cm) = 1/100 of a meter = 10 millimeters (mm) 1 meter (m) = 100 centimeters (cm)
Weight: Basic unit = gram 1 milligram (mg) = 1,000 micrograms (µg or mcg) = 1/1,000 of a gram (g) 1 gram (g) = 1,000 milligrams (mg) 1 kilogram (kg) = 1,000 grams (g)
Volume: Basic unit = liter 1 milliliter (mL) = 1/1,000 of a Liter = 1,000 microliters (µl) 1 liter (L) = 1,000 milliliters (mL)

> **Tip:** 1 milliliter (mL) is equivalent to 1 cubic centimeter (cc).

EXAMPLE

Converting Grams to Milligrams

42.3 g = _____ mg

Step 1: Determine the number of "space" between the two units of measure.

From grams to milligrams there are three spaces. Note the direction from gram to milligram is to the RIGHT.

Step 2: Move the decimal that number of spaces in the appropriate direction.

Move the decimal three places to the RIGHT. When moving a decimal where no number exists, simply add zeros.

$$42.3g = 42.\underset{1\ 2\ 3}{\underline{300}} = 42,300 \text{ mg}$$

Therefore, 42.3 g equals 42,300 mg.

Tip: Use this tool to easily convert between metric measurements.

Metric Prefix:	k	h	d	b	d	c	m	–	–	mc or μ
		← 3 Spaces →			← 3 Spaces →		← 3 Spaces →			
# of Spaces:	3	2	1		1	2	3	1	2	3

Remember that "b" stands for the base units of meters, liters or grams.

EXAMPLE

Converting Milligrams to Grams

1,430 mg = _____ g

Step 1: Determine the number of "space" between the two units of measure.

From milligrams to grams, there are three spaces. Note the direction from milligram to gram is to the LEFT.

Step 2: Move the decimal that number of spaces in the appropriate direction.

Move the decimal three places to the LEFT.

1,430 mg = 1430. = 1.43 g
      3 2 1

Therefore, 1,430 mg equals 1.43 g.

EXAMPLE
Converting Milligrams to Micrograms

2.8 mg = _____ mcg

Step 1: Determine the number of "space" between the two units of measure.

From milligrams to micrograms, there are three spaces. Note the direction from milligrams to micrograms is to the RIGHT.

Step 2: Move the decimal that number of spaces in the appropriate direction.

Move the decimal three places to the RIGHT. Remember, when moving a decimal where no number exists, simply add zeros.

2.8 mg = 2.800 mcg = 2,800 mcg
         1 2 3

Therefore, 2.8 mg equals 2,800 mcg.

EXAMPLE
Converting Liters to Milliliters

0.8 L = _____ mL

Step 1: Determine the number of "space" between the two units of measure.

From liters to milliliters, there are three spaces. Note the direction from liters to milliliters is to the RIGHT.

Step 2: Move the decimal that number of spaces in the appropriate direction.

Move the decimal three places to the RIGHT. When moving a decimal where no number exists, simply add zeros.

0.8 L = 0.800 = 800 mL

Therefore, 0.8 L equals 800 mL.

EXAMPLE
Converting Centimeters to Meters

3,600 cm = _____ m

Step 1: Determine the number of "space" between the two units of measure.

From centimeters to meters, there are two spaces. Note the direction from centimeters to meters is to the LEFT.

Step 2: Move the decimal that number of spaces in the appropriate direction.

Move the decimal two places to the LEFT. Remember, when moving a decimal where no number exists, just add zeros.

3,600 cm =3600.= 36 m

Therefore, 3,600 cm equals 36 m.

Most of the conversions used in a health care setting are done between kilograms (kg) and grams (g), grams (g) and milligrams (mg), milligrams (mg) and micrograms (mcg or µg), meters (m) and centimeters (cm), and liters (L) and milliliters (mL). Once these are practiced, converting between units will feel natural. Practice making the conversion by moving the decimal from one unit to another. Use a pencil to draw a "U" as you count the spaces. Start at the existing decimal and move to the right or left of each metric unit, depending on the conversion.

The Apothecary System

An apothecary is a pharmacist or someone who sells medications. This provides a key to remember how the system is most commonly used. Health care practitioners use apothecary measurements when writing prescriptions and to designate drug dosages for some of the medications that have existed for years.

The apothecary system is a system of weight and liquid measures. The basic apothecary solid (weight) measure is the grain (gr), while the basic fluid (volume) measure is the minim (♏ or ♏). It is important to note that the apothecary system does not include a length measurement.

> **Tip:** The abbreviation for grain is "gr" and the abbreviation for gram is "g"—be sure not to confuse the two.

The units of measure in the apothecary system have no simple relationship to each other; one must simply memorize this system to be able to use it. Tables 3 and 4 have been designed to simplify memorization and explain the relationship between the different units. When converting measures, if what you are converting is to a smaller measure (to the right in the table), you will use multiplication to solve. If what you are converting is to a larger measure (to the left in the table), you will use division to solve.

Table 3
Apothecary Weight Conversions

Pounds (℔)	Ounces (℥)	Drams or Drachms (ʒ)	Scruples (℈)	Grains (gr)
1 =	12 =	96 =	288 =	5,760
	1 =	8 =	24 =	480
		1 =	3 =	60
			1 =	20

Table 4
Apothecary Volume Conversions

Gallons (gal)	Quarts (qt)	Pints (pt)	Fluid Ounces (f℥)	Fluid Drams (f ʒ)	Minims (♏ or ♏)
1 =	4 =	8 =	128 =	1,024 =	61,440
	1 =	2 =	32 =	256 =	15,360
		1 =	16 =	128 =	7,680
			1 =	8 =	480
				1 =	60

> **Tip:** The apothecary pound is equal to 12 ounces, whereas the household pound is equal to 16 ounces.

EXAMPLE
Converting Apothecary Pounds to Ounces

1.5 pounds (℔) = _____ ounces (℥)

Step 1: Use the apothecary weight chart to determine the conversion between the two measures.

Using the apothecary weight chart, one can see each pound is equal to 12 ounces.

Step 2: Use multiplication to solve.

1.5 pounds x 12 ounces/pound =

1.5 ~~pounds~~ x 12 ounces/~~pound~~ =

1.5 x 12 ounces = 18 ounces

Therefore, 1.5 pounds (℔) equals 18 ounces (℥).

EXAMPLE
Converting Apothecary Grains to Drams

240 grains (gr) = _____ drams (ʒ)

Step 1: Use the apothecary weight chart to determine the conversion between the two measures.

Using the apothecary weight chart, one can see every dram contains 60 grains.

Step 2: Use division to solve. (Remember to consider the division rules of fractions when solving the problem.)

240 grains (gr) ÷ 60 grains/dram =

$$240 \, \text{gr} \times \frac{1 \, \text{dram}}{60 \, \text{gr}} = \frac{240 \, \text{drams}}{60} = 4 \, \text{drams}$$

Therefore, 240 grains (gr) equals 4 drams (ʒ).

EXAMPLE

Converting Apothecary Fluid Ounces to Fluid Drams

10 fluid ounces (f℥) = _____ fluid drams (fℨ)

Step 1: Use the apothecary volume chart to determine the conversion between the two measures.

Using the apothecary volume chart, one can see each fluid ounce is equal to 8 fluid drams.

Step 2: Use multiplication to solve.

10 ounces x 8 drams/ounce =
10 ~~ounces~~ x 8 drams/~~ounce~~ =
10 x 8 drams = 80 drams

Therefore, 10 fluid ounces (f℥) equals 80 fluid drams (fℨ).

EXAMPLE

Converting Apothecary Pints to Gallons

16 pints (pt) = _____ gallons (gal)

Step 1: Use the apothecary volume chart to determine the conversion between the two measures.

Using the apothecary volume chart, one can see every gallon contains 8 pints.

Step 2: Use division to solve. (Remember to consider the division rules of fractions when solving the problem.)

16 pints (pt) ÷ 8 pints/gallon =

$$16 \text{ pints} \times \frac{1 \text{ gallon}}{8 \text{ pints}} = \frac{16 \text{ gallons}}{8} = 2 \text{ gallons}$$

Therefore, 16 pints (pt) equals 2 gallons (gal).

The Avoirdupois System

The avoirdupois system is the ordinary system of weights used in the United States, in which 16 ounces avoirdupois equals a pound. The avoirdupois system is used only for measuring weight. Its basic unit is also the grain (gr). In practice, the avoirdupois system is most commonly used to measure weight, while the apothecary system is most commonly used to measure volume.

The avoirdupois system of weight is often used in commercial sales when buying and selling drugs and chemicals. Use of this system may be found on bulk bottles of chemicals used for compounding medications. As technicians become more involved in the distributive functions of the pharmacy, including the compounding process, they must have an understanding of the avoirdupois system to ensure accurate measurements.

Common terms are used to describe units in both the apothecary and avoirdupois systems. Be sure to take note of the difference in symbols used for the two systems to ensure accurate conversions when performing calculations.

Table 5
Avoirdupois Weight Conversions

Pound (lb)	Ounce (oz)	Grains (gr)
1 =	16 =	7,000
	1 =	437.5

> **Tip:** The grain is the only unit of measurement which has a value common to the apothecary and avoirdupois systems of measuring weight. The other denominations bearing the same name have quite different values.

EXAMPLE
Converting Avoirdupois Pounds to Ounces

4.75 pounds (lb) = _____ ounces (oz)

Step 1: Use the avoirdupois weight chart to determine the conversion between the two measures.

Using the avoirdupois weight chart, one can see each pound is equal to 16 ounces.

Step 2: Use multiplication to solve.

4.75 lbs x 16 oz/lb

The lbs cancel each other out, so:

4.75 x 16 oz = 76 oz

Therefore, 4.75 pounds (lb) equal 76 ounces (oz).

EXAMPLE
Converting Avoirdupois Grains to Ounces

782 grains (gr) = _____ ounces (oz)

Step 1: Use the avoirdupois weight chart to determine the conversion between the two measures.

Using the avoirdupois weight chart, one can see every ounce contains 437.5 grains.

Step 2: Use division to solve. (Remember to consider the division rules of fractions when solving the problem.)

$782 \text{ gr} \div 437.5 \text{ gr/oz} =$

$$782 \text{ gr} \times \frac{1 \text{ oz}}{437.5 \text{ gr}} = \frac{782 \text{ oz}}{437.5} = 1.7874 \text{ oz}$$

Therefore, 782 grains (gr) equals 1.79 ounces (oz) when rounded to two decimal places.

The apothecary and avoirdupois systems are still utilized in the practice of pharmacy. To determine the appropriate use for each system, one should keep in mind that the pharmacist may buy and sell bulk chemicals and drugs using the avoirdupois system of weight measurements. However, when compounding prescriptions, the pharmacist may employ the apothecary system of weight and volume to measure ingredients.

The Household Measurement System

The household system is the most commonly used system of measuring liquids in outpatient settings. Utensils that can be commonly found in any standard kitchen (i.e., teaspoons, tablespoons, etc.) are the equipment used to measure liquids.

The household system of measurement has no real scientific basis. It was established to provide a method of measurement that a patient could easily perform while measuring medications at home. This need for a simple and accurate method for measuring led to the development of household equivalents. It is important to be able to convert metric, apothecary or avoirdupois units to household measures, because most patients will be more familiar with these household measures and the devices used to measure them than with the other measurement systems.

Medication directions must be written in a manner that is understood by the patient to ensure the medication is measured and administered properly. The pharmacy technician must be able to convert any measurement system to a common household system when preparing prescriptions to be dispensed to a patient. The prescription label must include directions that will be clear to the patient, including what volume of medication to take when liquid preparations are dispensed.

Table 6 includes common household measurements and equivalent metric measures used in pharmacy practice.

Table 6
Common Household Measurements with Metric Equivalents

Measurement Unit	Equivalent in Household System	Equivalent(s) in a Metric System
1 teaspoonful (tsp or t) =		5 mL
1 tablespoonful (tbs or T) =	3 tsp =	15 mL
1 fluid ounce (fl oz) =	2 tbs =	30 mL
1 glassful/cupful =	8 fl oz =	240 mL
1 pint (pt) =	2 cups =	473 mL (commonly rounded to 480 mL)
1 quart (qt) =	2 pt =	946 mL (commonly rounded to 1 L)
1 gallon (gal) =	4 qt =	3,785 mL

EXAMPLE
Converting Fluid Ounces to Milliliters

16 fluid ounces (fl oz) = _____ milliliters (mL)

Step 1: Use the household measurements chart to determine the conversion factor.

Using the chart, 1 fluid ounce = 30 milliliters

Step 2: Use proportions or multiplication to solve.

To convert fluid ounces to milliliters, one can simply multiply by 30 or solve the problem using proportions and the conversion factor of 1 fluid ounce = 30 milliliters, as follows.

$$\frac{1 \text{ oz}}{16 \text{ oz}} = \frac{30 \text{ mL}}{Z \text{ mL}}$$

Z mL = 16 x 30

Z = 480 mL

Therefore, 16 fluid ounces (fl oz) equals 480 milliliters (mL).

EXAMPLE
Converting Milliliters to Tablespoons

45 mL = _____ tbs

Step 1: Use the household measurements chart to determine the conversion factor.

Using the chart, 15 milliliters = 1 tablespoon

Step 2: Use proportions or multiplication to solve.

To convert milliliters to tablespoons, one can simply divide by 15 or solve the problem using proportions and the conversion factor 15 milliliters = 1 tablespoon, as follows.

$$\frac{1 \text{ tbs}}{Z \text{ tbs}} = \frac{15 \text{ mL}}{45 \text{ mL}}$$

15 Z = 45

$$\frac{\cancel{15}Z}{\cancel{15}} = \frac{45}{15}$$

Z = 3

Therefore, 45 milliliters (mL) equals 3 tablespoons (tbs).

Conversions Between Systems

A quantity called for in one system may have to be "translated" to another system. This translation is called **conversion**. Conversion is frequently required because multiple measurement systems are used in pharmacy practice. Since metric, avoirdupois (weight), U.S. liquid measure (volume) and apothecary (volume and weight) systems of measurement are all different, conversions are always required when quantities must be compared. Inches may not be added to meters, pounds may not be subtracted from kilograms and tablespoons may not be added to minims. When working with multiple measurement systems, one must convert to a single system (usually the metric system) before proceeding with mathematical calculations. These types of calculations are often required when compounding medications. It is important to understand that these conversions are roughly equivalent, but are not exact conversions. A general rule in pharmacy practice suggests one should use between a two- and three-figure accuracy when rounding calculations.

To convert between measurement systems, simply set up a proportion, using fractions, and multiply the fractions to find the correct answer.

Table 7

Apothecary System with Metric Equivalents

Apothecary Fluid Measure (Volume)

Measurement Unit	Equivalent in System	Metric Equivalent
1 minim (℩)		0.0626 mL
1 fluid dram (f℥)	60 ℩	3.696 mL
1 fluid ounce (f℥)	8 f℥	29.573 mL or 29.57 mL
1 pint (pt)	16 f℥	473 mL or 0.473 L
1 quart (qt)	2 pt or 32 f℥	946.4 mL or 0.9464 L
1 gallon (gal)	4 qt or 8 pt	3,785 mL or 3.785 L

Apothecary Dry or Solid Measure (Weight)

Measurement Unit	Equivalent in System	Metric Equivalent
1 grain (gr)		0.065 g or 65 mg
1 scruple (℈)	20 gr	1.296 g
1 drachm or dram (℥)	3 ℈ or 60 gr	3.887 g
1 ounce (℥)	8 ℥ or 480 gr	31.103 g
1 pound (℔)	12 ℥ or 5,760 gr	373 g or 0.373 kg

Table 8
Avoirdupois System with Metric Equivalents

Avoirdupois Dry or Solid Measure (Weight)

Measurement Unit	Equivalent in System	Metric Equivalent
1 grain (gr)		0.0648 g or 65 mg
1 ounce (oz)	437.5 gr	28.35 g
1 pound (lb)	16 oz or 7,000 gr	454 g or 0.454 kg

Table 9
Commonly Used Conversions

Measurement	Equivalent
1 inch (in) =	2.54 centimeters (cm)
1 meter (m) =	39.4 inch (in)
1 grain (gr) =	65 milligram (mg)
1 gram (g) =	15 grain (gr)
1 kilogram (kg) =	2.2 pounds (lb)
1 ounce (oz) =	30 milliliter (mL)

EXAMPLE
Converting Fluid Ounces to Milliliters

6 fluid ounces (f℥) = _____ milliliters (mL)

Step 1: Determine conversion factor.

The conversion factor is 1 fluid ounce = 29.57 milliliters.

Step 2: Use multiplication or proportions to solve.

To convert fluid ounces to milliliters, one can simply multiply by 29.57 or solve the problem using proportions and the conversion factor of 1 fluid ounce = 29.57 milliliters.

$$\frac{1 \text{ f℥}}{6 \text{ f℥}} = \frac{29.57 \text{ mL}}{Z \text{ mL}}$$

Z mL = 6 × 29.57

Z = 177.42 mL

Therefore, 6 fluid ounces equals 177.42 mL.

EXAMPLE
Converting Millimeters to Inches

569 millimeters (mm) = _____ inches (in)

Step 1: Determine the conversion factor.

1 inch equals 2.54 centimeters. Therefore, in this problem, millimeters must first be converted to centimeters.

There are 10 millimeters per 1 centimeter.

569 mm ÷ 10 mm/cm

$$569 \text{ mm} \times \frac{\text{cm}}{10 \text{ mm}} = \frac{569 \text{ cm}}{10} = 56.9 \text{ cm}$$

Step 2: Use division or proportions to solve.

To convert centimeters to inches one can simply divide by 2.54 or solve the problem using proportions and the conversion factor of 1 inch = 2.54 centimeters.

$$\frac{1 \text{ in}}{Z \text{ in}} = \frac{2.54 \text{ cm}}{56.9 \text{ cm}}$$

56.9 = 2.54 Z

$$\frac{56.9}{2.54} = Z$$

Z = 22.40157 inches, rounded to 22.4 inches

Therefore, 569 millimeters equals 22.4 inches.

EXAMPLE

Converting Grams to Grains

4.5 grams (g) = _____ grains (gr)

Step 1: Determine conversion factor.

The conversion factor is 1 gram = 15 grains.

Step 2: Use multiplication or proportions to solve.

To convert grams to grains one can simply multiply by 15 grains or solve the problem using proportions and the conversion factor of 1 gram = 15 grains.

$$\frac{1 \text{ g}}{4.5 \text{ g}} = \frac{15 \text{ gr}}{Z \text{ gr}}$$

Z gr = 4.5 x 15

Z = 67.5 grains

Therefore, 4.5 grams equals 67.5 grains.

Conclusion

Though the metric system is commonly used in pharmacy practice, other measurement systems, such as apothecary, avoirdupois and household, may be encountered by pharmacy technicians. It is important for technicians to be able to recognize and work with these systems in order to be effective in their job responsibilities.

Chapter 3
PRACTICE PROBLEMS

1. What is the metric system's basic unit of measure for volume?
   a. Liter
   b. Gram
   c. Grain
   d. Pint

2. What is the metric system's basic unit of measure for length?
   a. Scruple
   b. Minim
   c. Meter
   d. Mile

3. What is the metric system's basic unit of measure for weight?
   a. Pound
   b. Ounce
   c. Gram
   d. Quart

4. The prefix "deci" represents what value?
   a. 1,000
   b. 100
   c. 10
   d. 0.1

5. The prefix "micro" has what value?
   a. One hundredth
   b. One thousand
   c. One millionth
   d. One hundred

6. What prefix and symbol represent one hundred?
   a. Kilo, k
   b. Hecto, h
   c. Milli, m
   d. Centi, c

7. How many millimeters are in 3 centimeters?
    a. 3
    b. 30
    c. 300
    d. 3,000

8. Using the apothecary system, how many ounces are in a pound?
    a. 12
    b. 14
    c. 16
    d. 20

9. What is the basic apothecary unit of measure for weight?
    a. Pound
    b. Ounce
    c. Grain
    d. Minim

10. What is the basic apothecary unit of measure for volume?
    a. Pint
    b. Dram
    c. Minim
    d. Ounce

11. How many grains does an avoirdupois pound equal?
    a. 5,000
    b. 6,000
    c. 7,000
    d. 8,000

12. One tablespoon equals how many milliliters?
    a. 15
    b. 30
    c. 45
    d. 60

13. One quart equals how many cups?
    a. 2
    b. 3
    c. 4
    d. 5

14. True or False: The ounce measure in the avoirdupois and apothecary systems have two different values.

15. One inch equals how many centimeters?
    a. 1.43
    b. 2.15
    c. 2.54
    d. 3.09

Convert the following units of measure.

16. 56 g = _____ mg
     a. 5.6
     b. 560
     c. 5,600
     d. 56,000

17. 4,670 mg = _____ g
     a. 4.67
     b. 46.7
     c. 467
     d. 46,700

18. 1.2 mg = _____ mcg
     a. 12
     b. 120
     c. 1,200
     d. 12,000

19. 0.3 L = _____ mL
     a. 3
     b. 30
     c. 300
     d. 3,000

20. 5,800 cm = _____ m
     a. 580
     b. 58
     c. 5.8
     d. 0.58

21. 2.3 ℔ = _____ ℨ
     a. 27.6
     b. 32.5
     c. 28.4
     d. 36.8

22. 420 gr = _____ ℨ
     a. 2.4
     b. 7
     c. 25,200
     d. 42,000

23. 15 f℥ = _____ f℥
     a. 1.875
     b. 120
     c. 45
     d. 360

24. 82 pt = _____ gal
    a. 27.3
    b. 13.6
    c. 12
    d. 10.25

25. 7.77 lb = _____ oz
    a. 62.16
    b. 93.24
    c. 108.78
    d. 124.32

26. 562 gr = _____ oz
    a. 1.28
    b. 1.17
    c. 9.37
    d. 7.03

27. 6.2 L = _____ mL
    a. 62
    b. 620
    c. 6,200
    d. 620,000

28. 327 mL = _____ L
    a. 3.27
    b. 3270
    c. 32.7
    d. 0.327

29. 8.91 mm = _____ μm
    a. 89.1
    b. 89,100
    c. 8,910
    d. 891

30. 45 mL = _____ L
    a. 4.5
    b. 0.45
    c. 0.045
    d. 0.0045

31. 1.47 ℔ = _____ ℨ
    a. 17.64
    b. 14.7
    c. 5
    d. 23.52

32. 3,960 gr = _____ ʒ
    a. 198
    b. 13.75
    c. 66
    d. 660

33. 73 fʒ = _____ qt
    a. 0.29
    b. 9.13
    c. 0.57
    d. 4,380

34. 11 gal = _____ fʒ
    a. 704
    b. 176
    c. 88
    d. 1,408

35. 6 oz = _____ gr
    a. 187
    b. 2,625
    c. 3,500
    d. 720

36. 18 qt = _____ pt
    a. 24
    b. 30
    c. 48
    d. 36

37. 7 ʒ = _____ gr
    a. 9,600
    b. 3,360
    c. 24
    d. 217.72

38. 3,660 ♏ = _____ fʒ
    a. 61
    b. 458
    c. 24
    d. 229

39. 7,000 gr = _____ oz
    a. 22
    b. 424
    c. 16
    d. 1,024

40. 5 pt = _____ f℥
    a. 96
    b. 640
    c. 48
    d. 80

41. 14 tsp = _____ mL
    a. 28
    b. 140
    c. 30
    d. 70

42. 255 lb = _____ kg (use avoirdupois system)
    a. 137.4
    b. 169.1
    c. 115.9
    d. 267.3

43. 734 mg = _____ gr
    a. 11.29
    b. 14.25
    c. 6.34
    d. 8.95

44. 6 qt = _____ L
    a. 12
    b. 3.567
    c. 5.676
    d. 8.6576

45. 13 g = _____ gr (use apothecary conversion)
    a. 107.69
    b. 200
    c. 118.45
    d. 20.7

46. 4,665.5 g = _____ ℥
    a. 150
    b. 200
    c. 115
    d. 100

47. 9 gr = _____ mg
    a. 540
    b. 630
    c. 785
    d. 585

48. 540 mL = _____ oz
    a. 16
    b. 24
    c. 18
    d. 32

49. 22 fʒ = _____ mL
    a. 70.5
    b. 81.3
    c. 62.4
    d. 66.5

50. 14 cups = _____ mL
    a. 3,120
    b. 2,340
    c. 3,360
    d. 1,820

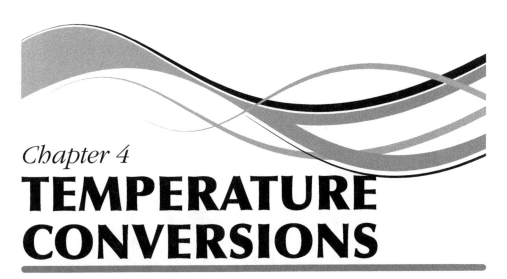

Chapter 4
TEMPERATURE CONVERSIONS

By   Theresa A. Mozug, CPhT, B.S.
Amal A. Sobh, Pharm.D.

Learning Objectives

Upon completion of this chapter, a technician should be able to:
- identify the two systems used to measure temperature.
- learn which system is used most widely in the scientific community.
- determine the three formulas that can be used to convert between temperature measurement systems.

Introduction

Most of the world uses either the Fahrenheit or Celsius system to measure temperature. In the United States, Fahrenheit is most often used. Celsius temperature measurement is a component of the metric system, which is used by most other countries. Though the general population of the United States uses Fahrenheit to measure temperature, the scientific community uses the Celsius temperature scale. Therefore, it is essential that the pharmacy technician be able to convert between the two systems.

Temperature Measurement Systems

Both Fahrenheit and Celsius systems are based on the freezing and boiling points of water. The Celsius system is based upon the centigrade scale. Therefore, the freezing point of water is 0 °C and the boiling point is 100 °C. The freezing point of water in the Fahrenheit system is 32 °F and the boiling point is 212 °F.

The numerical relationship of Celsius to Fahrenheit is:

F temperature = (1.8 or $\frac{9}{5}$ x the number of degrees Celsius) + 32

This formula can be simplified into three possible equations (or formulas) that may be used to convert temperatures between the two systems.

Formula #1

$9C = 5F - 160$

C = Degrees Celsius
F = Degrees Fahrenheit

When one of the values is given, the equation may be used to solve for the unknown value.

EXAMPLE
Converting Degrees Fahrenheit (°F) to Degrees Celsius (°C) Using Formula #1

What is the temperature in degrees Celsius when degrees Fahrenheit is 43?

Step 1: Insert known value (degrees Fahrenheit) into Formula #1 and solve.

$9C = 5F - 160$

$9C = (5 \times 43) - 160$

$9C = 215 - 160$

$9C = 55$

$$\frac{9C}{9} = \frac{55}{9}$$

$C = 6.1 \ °C$

Therefore, 43 °F is equal to 6.1 °C.

Formula #2 for converting between the two temperature systems can be written in two formats as follows:

Format (a):   **Format (b):**

$C = (F - 32) \div 1.8$ **OR** $F = (C \times 1.8) + 32$

EXAMPLE
Converting Degrees Fahrenheit to Degrees Celsius Using Formula #2a

What is the temperature in degrees Celsius when degrees Fahrenheit is 43?

Step 1: Insert the known value (degrees Fahrenheit) into Formula #2a and solve.

$C = (F - 32) \div 1.8$

$C = (43 - 32) \div 1.8$

$C = 11 \div 1.8$

$C = 6.1 \,°C$

Therefore, 43 °F is equal to 6.1 °C.

EXAMPLE
Converting Degrees Celsius to Degrees Fahrenheit Using Formula #2b

What is the temperature in degrees Fahrenheit when degrees Celsius is 6.1?

Step 1: Insert the known value (degrees Celsius) into the Formula #2b and solve.

$F = (C \times 1.8) + 32$

$F = (6.1 \times 1.8) + 32$

$F = 10.98 + 32$

$F = 42.98$ or 43 °F

Therefore, 6.1 °C is equal to 43 °F

Formula #3 is the final formula that is used for temperature conversions, which can also be written in two formats as follows:

Format (a):   **Format (b):**

$$C = (F - 32) \times \frac{5}{9} \quad \textbf{OR} \quad F = \left(C \times \frac{9}{5} \right) + 32$$

EXAMPLE

Converting Degrees Fahrenheit to Degrees Celsius Using Formula #3a

What is the temperature in degrees Celsius when degrees Fahrenheit is 43?

Step 1: Insert the known value (degrees Fahrenheit) into Formula #3a and solve.

$$C = (F - 32) \times \frac{5}{9}$$

$$C = (43 - 32) \times \frac{5}{9}$$

$$C = 11 \times \frac{5}{9}$$

$$C = \left(\frac{11 \times 5}{9}\right)$$

$$C = \frac{55}{9}$$

$$C = 6.1\,°C$$

Therefore, 43 °F is equal to 6.1 °C.

EXAMPLE

Converting Degrees Celsius to Degrees Fahrenheit Using Formula #3b

What is the temperature in degrees Fahrenheit when degrees Celsius is 6.1?

Step 1: Insert the known value (degrees Celsius) into Formula #3b and solve.

$$F = \left(C \times \frac{9}{5}\right) + 32$$

$$F = \left(6.1 \times \frac{9}{5}\right) + 32$$

$$F = \left(\frac{6.1 \times 9}{5}\right) + 32$$

$$F = \frac{54.9}{5} + 32$$

$$F = 10.98 + 32$$

$$F = 42.98 \text{ or } 43°F$$

Therefore, 6.1 °C is equal to 43°F

Tip: Use any of the three formulas for any conversion problem. The answer will be the same regardless of which formula is used.

NOTE: Sometimes negative numbers may figure into the equation because temperatures will drop below zero. An example follows.

EXAMPLE
Converting Degrees Fahrenheit to Degrees Celsius When a Negative Number is Involved

What is the temperature in degrees Celsius when degrees Fahrenheit is 22?

Use the following formula to solve for the unknown, which in this case, is degrees Celsius.

$$5F - 160 = 9C$$

Step 1: Insert the known value (degrees Fahrenheit) into the equation and solve.

$$(5 \times 22) - 160 = 9C$$

$$110 - 160 = 9C$$

$$-50 = 9C$$

$$\frac{-50}{9} = \frac{9C}{9}$$

$$C = -5.55°C$$

Therefore, 22 °F is equal to -5.6 °C.

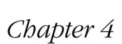

Chapter 4

PRACTICE PROBLEMS

For problems 1-5, convert the Fahrenheit temperatures to Celsius using Formula #1. Round answers to the nearest tenth.

> *Formula #1:*
> 9C = 5F – 160, where C is degrees Celsius and F is degrees Fahrenheit

1. 13 °F

2. 98 °F

3. 64 °F

4. 71 °F

5. 102 °F

For problems 6-10, convert the following Celsius temperatures to Fahrenheit using Formula #1. Round answers to the nearest tenth.

6. 50 °C

7. 25 °C

8. 2 °C

9. 31 °C

10. 15 °C

For problems 11-20, convert the following Fahrenheit temperatures to Celsius using Formula #2a. Round answers to the nearest tenth.

> *Formula #2a:*
> C = (F – 32) ÷ 1.8, where C is degrees Celsius and F is degrees Fahrenheit

11. 66 °F

12. 49 °F

13. -7 °F

14. 29 °F

15. 14 °F

16. 34 °F

17. 78 °F

18. 55 °F

19. 82 °F

20. 65 °F

For problems 21-30, convert the following Celsius temperatures to Fahrenheit using Formula #2b. Round answers to the nearest tenth.

Formula #2b:

F = (C x 1.8) + 32, where C is degrees Celsius and F is degrees Fahrenheit

21. 3 °C

22. -15 °C

23. 16 °C

24. 28 °C

25. 10 °C

26. 11 °C

27. 8 °C

28. 22 °C

29. 42 °C

30. 18 °C

For problems 31-40, convert the following Fahrenheit temperatures to Celsius using Formula #3a. Round answers to the nearest tenth.

Formula #3a:

$$C = (F - 32) \times \frac{5}{9}$$, where C is degrees Celsius and F is degrees Fahrenheit

31. 143 °F

32. 0 °F

33. 44 °F

34. 26 °F

35. 15 °F

36. 156 °F

37. 42 °F

38. 63 °F

39. 57 °F

40. 18 °F

For problems 41-50, convert the following Celsius temperatures to Fahrenheit using Formula #3b. Round answers to the nearest tenth.

Formula #3b:

$$F = \left(C \times \frac{9}{5}\right) + 32 \text{, where C is degrees Celsius and F is degrees Fahrenheit}$$

41. 9 °C

42. 33° C

43. -6 °C

44. 42 °C

45. 20 °C

46. 31 °C

47. 8 °C

48. 22 °C

49. 42 °C

50. -5 °C

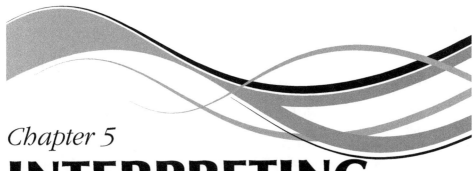

Chapter 5
INTERPRETING MEDICATION ORDERS

By Derek J. Quinn, Pharm.D.

Learning Objectives

Upon completion of this chapter, the technician should be able to:
- interpret standard medical abbreviations used in medication orders (prescriptions).
- convert between Roman numerals and Arabic numerals.
- discuss common elements of outpatient and inpatient medication/device orders.
- verify the check digit of a Drug Enforcement Agency (DEA) registration number.
- verify the check digit of a National Provider Identifier (NPI).

Introduction

Patients may need any number of medications and devices as part of managing their disease states. Most medications and many devices (and the supplies for those devices) are ordered by prescribers on a prescription. In the inpatient setting, prescriptions are commonly referred to as medication orders. Most prescriptions are written for items that require a prescription; however, prescriptions may also be written for items that are medically necessary for a patient but that don't require a prescription (i.e., over-the-counter (OTC) drugs). This chapter will expose a technician to the common ways in which prescriptions are transmitted from the prescriber, through a pharmacy to a patient, and to some of the skills necessary to be an effective part of this transmission process.

Medical Abbreviations

Most abbreviations used in medicine come from Latin, though some are from Greek, French, German and other languages. Many new abbreviations come from English, but the use of Latin is still alive and well in medical jargon. Technicians must be able to convert freely between the common abbreviations and the English interpretation of those abbreviations. Abbreviation misinterpretation can be a source for medications errors, as many common abbreviations are very close to other common abbreviations. Some patient safety organizations and accrediting groups have lists of banned abbreviations; an abbreviation is usually considered banned if it is commonly involved in medication errors or is more likely to cause medication errors because it looks or sounds like another abbreviation.

The following chart is a list of common abbreviations seen on prescriptions, the Latin that the abbreviation is based upon (when appropriate) and the English interpretation of the abbreviation that will be used when typing a prescription label for a patient. Abbreviations for common measurements (e.g., "mL") and elements on the periodic table (e.g., FeSO4) appear elsewhere and are not included in this list. This list is not meant to be complete; rather, it is a place to begin.

Common Pharmacy Abbreviations

Abbreviation	Full Latin Text	English Interpretation
AC (a.c.)	Ante Cibum	before a meal or meals
CAUTION AD (a.d.)	Auris Dextra	right ear
APAP		N-acetyl-p-aminophenol (the active component in acetaminophen)
AQ (a.q.)	Aqua	water
CAUTION AS (a.s.)	Auris Sinistra	left ear
ASA		Acetylsalicylic Acid (aspirin)
CAUTION AU (a.u.)	Auris Utraque	both ears
BID	Bis In Die	twice daily
BIW		twice weekly
BSA		Body Surface Area
c or c/	Cum	with
cc	Cum Cibo	with food
CAUTION cc		Cubic Centimeter
CR		Controlled Release
D5W		Dextrose 5% in Water

Abbreviation	Full Latin Text	English Interpretation
D5NS		Dextrose 5% in Normal Saline
DAW (d.a.w.)		Dispense As Written
◆ d/c or DC		DisContinue
EC		Enteric-Coated
ER		Extended Release
FBS		Fasting Blood Sugar
gtt or gtts	Gutta (plural = Guttae)	Drop(s)
HCTZ		Hydrochlorothiazide
HS (h.s.)	Hora Somni	At bedtime
HTN		Hypertension (high blood pressure)
IEN or EN		In Each Nostril
IM		Intramuscular (into the muscle)
IR		Immediate Release
IV		Itravenous (into the vein)
IVP		Intravenous Push
IVPB		Intravenous Piggyback
mEq		Milli-Equivalent
MVI		Multi-Vitamin
noc or noct	Nocte	at night
NS		Normal Saline (0.9% NaCl)
1/2NS		Half (1/2) Normal Saline (0.45% NaCl)
◆ OD (o.d.)	Oculus Dexter	right eye
ODT		Orally-Disintegrating Tablet
◆ OS (o.s.)	Oculus Sinister	left eye
◆ OU (o.u.)	Oculus Utraque	both eyes
Per	Per	through

Abbreviation	Full Latin Text	English Interpretation
PC (p.c.)	**P**ost **C**ibum (plural = Post Cibos)	after a meal or meals
PRN	**P**ro **Re N**ata	as needed
PRN/Anx or P/Anx or prnax		as needed for anxiety
PRN/NV or PNV or P/NV		as needed for nausea and vomiting
PRN/P or P/P		as needed for pain
PO (p.o.)	**P**er **O**s	by mouth
PR (p.r.)		through the rectum
PV (p.v.)		through the vagina
Q	**Q**uaque	every
QAM	**Q**uaque (die) **A**nte **M**eridiem	every day, in the morning
◆CAUTION QD (q.d.)	**Q**uaque **D**ie	(once) every day
QH (q.h.)	**Q**uaque **H**ora	every hour
◆CAUTION QHS (q.h.s.)	**Q**uaque (die) **H**ora **S**omnis	every day, at bedtime
QID (q.i.d.)	**Q**uater **I**n **D**ie	four times each day
QOD (q.o.d.)		every other day
QPM	**Q**uaque (die) **P**ost **M**eridiem	every day, in the evening
Q4h		every four hours
Q6h		every six hours
Q4/6h		every four to six hours
QS (q.s.)	**Q**uantum **S**ufficiat	**Q**uantity **S**ufficient
s or s/	**S**ine	without
SA		**S**ustained **A**ction
◆CAUTION SC, SubQ, SQ		**S**ub**C**utaneous (below the skin)
Sig		write on label / post this sign

Abbreviation	Full Latin Text	English Interpretation
SL		**S**ub**L**ingual (under the tongue)
SR		**S**ustained **R**elease
Stat	**Stat**im	immediately!
†		one
††		two
†††		three
TID	**T**er **I**n **D**ie	three times daily
TIW		three times weekly
TPN		**T**otal **P**arenteral (non-oral) **N**utrition
UD or UAD or UtD or UtDict	**U**t **D**ictum	as directed
XL		Extended Release
XR		Extended **R**elease

 Some of the abbreviations in this list have been reported to the Institute for Safe Medication Practices (ISMP) as being frequently misinterpreted and involved in harmful medication errors. They are provided here because, unfortunately, they are still often used, and pharmacy technicians must be diligent to make sure they correctly understand a prescription. Do not use these abbreviations at your pharmacy in communicating with other medical professionals. Be sure to check the ISMP's List of Error-Prone Abbreviations, Symbols and Dose Designations at www.ismp.org.

EXAMPLE
Interpreting Abbreviations on a Prescription

Interpret this typical prescription.

Patient: Ms. Betty Sunshine (DOB: 1/11/1950)
Hydrocodone / Acetaminophen 5 mg/500 mg
Sig: †/†† PO Q4/6H P/P
Disp #40 (Forty) Ref: 2
Dr. Ortho Breaker
Written: 1/15/2010

This should be interpreted as follows:
Give Ms. Betty Sunshine (Date of Birth: 1/11/1950) hydrocodone/acetaminophen 5 mg/500 mg tablets labeled with directions of "Take one or two tablets, by mouth, every four to six hours as needed for pain." Dispense 40 tablets and label with two refills from Dr. Ortho Breaker.

To break down the directions (sig):
†/†† means "take one or two tablets"
PO means "by mouth"
Q4/6H means "every four to six hours"
P/P means "as needed for pain"

Roman Numerals

Medicine also uses the Latin numbering system (known as Roman numerals) on occasion. A technician must be able to fluidly convert between Roman numerals (e.g., i, ii, iii, iv) and Arabic numerals (e.g., 1, 2, 3, 4). When Roman numerals are used on prescriptions, a technician must convert the Roman numeral into an Arabic numeral for the patient, as many patients are unfamiliar with Roman numerals. The following chart gives the Roman numeral and the Arabic numeral.

Roman Numeral	Arabic Numeral
I or i	1 (one)
V or v	5 (five)
X or x	10 (ten)
L	50 (fifty)
C	100 (one hundred)
D	500 (five hundred)
M	1,000 (one thousand)

Using these Roman numeral bases as a starting point, any number larger than one can be written using Roman numerals (traditionally, there is no zero in Roman numerals). To express the values between two of the bases (e.g., i and v), multiple Roman numerals are placed next to each other, and they are either added or subtracted from one another. Generally, four of the same base units do not appear together (e.g., iiii is not used). When interpreting a longer number represented by Roman numerals, the highest number will be on the left and the smallest number on the right (e.g., in MXI [1,011], the M [1,000] comes to the left of the XI [11]). When a SMALLER numeral comes BEFORE a larger base, the smaller numeral is subtracted from the larger base (e.g., IX = 10 – 1 = 9); when a LARGER numeral comes AFTER a larger base, the smaller numeral is added to the larger base (e.g., VII = 5 + 1 + 1 = 7).

When there are more than two Roman numerals strung together, the same rule applies—subtract when the left numeral in a pair is smaller than the right numeral and add when the right numeral is smaller than the left numeral. The only difference is that one must first find the highest value Roman numeral and separate everything that comes before it and everything that comes after it into two parts and deal with each part separately (e.g., CMVII, where M has the highest value, must be separated into C, M, and VII). First, determine the value of the part that was to the left of the highest value Roman numeral (e.g., C = 100). Second, determine the value of the part that was to the right of the highest value Roman numeral (e.g., VII = 5 + 1 + 1 = 7). Third, subtract the part that was to the left of the highest value Roman numeral from the highest value Roman numeral (e.g., M-C = 1,000 – 100 = 900) and add the part that was to the right of the highest value Roman numeral (e.g., add VII = 7 to 900). Therefore, CMVII = 907.

EXAMPLE

Converting Roman Numerals to Arabic Numerals

Convert DCCCXLII to an Arabic numeral.

Step 1: Determine the highest value Roman numeral.

The highest value is D. D = 500

Step 2: Determine the value of any numerals to the left of the highest numeral.

There is nothing to the left of D.

Step 3: Determine the value of the numerals to the right of the highest numeral.

CCCXLII is to the right of the D. It equals:
1. CCC = 100 + 100 + 100 = 300
2. When a smaller numeral (X) comes before a larger base (L), the smaller numeral is subtracted from the larger. XL = 50 − 10 = 40
3. II = 1 + 1 = 2
4. 300 + 40 + 2 = 342

Step 4: Add the value in Step 3 to the highest numeral for the total value of the Roman numerals.

500 + 342 = 842

Therefore, DCCCXLII = 842.

Tip: When finding a value for a Roman numeral, determine the highest value numeral. Then if there is a number to the left, subtract. If there is a number to the right, add. Repeat with next highest numeral, etc., until all numerals are addressed.

EXAMPLE
Converting Roman Numerals to Arabic Numerals

Convert MCMXCIX to an Arabic numerals.

Step 1: Determine the highest value Roman numeral.

The highest value is M. M = 1,000

Step 2: Since there are two of the highest value numerals, start with determining the first numerals value.

The first M has nothing to the left of it, so its value is 1,000.

Step 3: Determine the value of the second, highest value numeral.

The second M has a C to the left of it.

C = 100

So, CM = 1,000 – 100 = 900

Step 4: Determine the value of the numerals to the right of the second, highest numeral.

XCIX is to the right of the MCM.
1. When a smaller numeral (X) comes before a larger base (C), the smaller numeral is subtracted from the larger. XC = 100 – 10 = 90
2. When a smaller numeral (I) comes before a larger base (X), the smaller numeral is subtracted from the larger. IX = 10 – 1 = 9
3. 90 + 9 = 99

Step 5: Add all of the calculated values for the total.

1,000 + 900 + 99 = 1,999

Therefore, MCMXCIX = 1,999.

Although conversion from Arabic numerals to Roman numerals rarely arises in practice, a technician must be able to convert freely back and forth.

EXAMPLE

Converting From Arabic Numerals to Roman Numerals

Convert 5,280 to a Roman numerals.

Step 1: Determine the highest value to convert.

The highest value is 5,000. 5,000 = MMMMM

Step 2: Determine the next value to the right of the highest value.

To the right of the 5,000 will be 200. 200 = CC

Step 3: Continue to repeat Step 2 until each digit in the Arabic numeral is converted.

To the right of the 200 will be 80. 80 = LXXX

Step 4: Put all of the values together from left to right.

MMMMMCCLXXX

Interpreting Common Orders

Although each state has its own laws for exactly what is required on a prescription or medication order, there are some commonalities that each prescription must have. The identity of the patient and prescriber must be sufficient to determine exactly for whom the order is written and who wrote the order. The patient's date of birth (DOB) is often listed on a prescription to help in identifying the patient. Prescribers, like pharmacies, have many different identifying numbers that can be used on a prescription to properly identify themselves. Later in this chapter, the Drug Enforcement Agency (DEA) Number and National Provider Identifier (NPI) will be discussed in detail; these are two of the numbers that prescribers can use to identify themselves on a prescription. Finally, the drug and how the drug is to be used and dispensed must be on every medication order.

All medication orders must include directions for the patient's use of the drug. Directions given to patients must not only be very specific, but they also must prevent misuse of medications by warning patients of potential pitfalls before they become problems. Nearly every outpatient pharmacy has a story of a patient who followed the all-too-unspecific directions on a label as step-by-step instructions and therefore didn't take the aluminum foil off of their rectal suppositories before inserting them. Ouch! These types of problems have resulted in some standard directions that are used when typing labels for certain products. Further, since directions always involve an action step, choosing the proper action verb is key to patients using medications as prescribed. A list of common verbs and when they are used is listed below. Note that for most adults, directions for oral medications begin with "take" as the person reading the directions will likely be the patient; however, for children and those with caregivers, it is usually appropriate to begin with "give" (e.g., Give one tablet, by mouth, at bedtime). Finally, it is recommended that a route of administration be given on every prescription label (e.g., by mouth, in the left eye, nasally). Always remember that a real person will be reading the directions you provide and will be using their medication exactly how they interpret what appears on the label. Think through how a medication could be misused and then adjust your typing practices to prevent that misuse.

Type of Drug	Verb for Use
Oral Solids (Tabs/Caps) and Liquids	Take/Give by Mouth
Nasal Sprays	Spray Nasally
Topicals	Apply to the Affected Area(s)
Suppositories	Unwrap and Insert
Inhalers	Inhale (puffs) by Mouth
Injectables	Inject (Subcutaneously or Intramuscularly)
Eye Drops / Ear Drops	Instill or Place into the Affected Eye(s)/Ear(s)

FOR EXAMPLE

Flonase® Nasal Spray "†† EN BID" would expand "Spray twice into each nostril twice daily"

Vagifem® Vaginal Tablets "† QHS" would expand "Insert one tablet vaginally at bedtime"

Advair® Diskus Inhaler "† BID" would expand "Inhale one puff, by mouth, twice daily"

Lovenox® 40 mg/0.4 mL "40 mg SQ Q12h" would expand "Inject one syringeful (40 mg) subcutaneously every twelve hours"

EXAMPLE
Reading a Properly Written Prescription

Patient: Grumpy Gus (DOB: 4/1/1965)

Date Written: 1/15/2013

Oxycodone / Acetaminophen 10 mg/325 mg
Sig: †/†† PO Q4/6H P/P
Disp #360 (three hundred sixty) Ref: 0 (zero)

Dr. I.D. Issues
DEA#: BD8031259
NPI: 6784527541

This prescription can be read as follows:
Give Grumpy Gus (Date of Birth April 1, 1965) oxy-codone/acetaminophen 10 mg/325 mg tablets with directions: Take one or two tablets, by mouth, every four to six hours as needed for pain. Dispense three hundred sixty tablets (360) without refills. Written by Dr. I.D. Issues with the DEA Number and NPI listed.

The above example prescription is for a tablet, which is easily measured by counting the units to be given (i.e., "give one or two tablet(s)"). When medications are given as liquids, a calibrated measuring device must be used by the patient to properly dose the drug being administered. Patients are never advised to use the silverware from their drawer to measure medications. Always be sure that the directions on the label match up with the markings on the measuring device that is going to be used; most dose cups/spoons come with both American standard units (e.g., teaspoons or ounces) and metric units (e.g., mL). Since the standard measurement unit of the scientific and health care communities is metric, it is preferred that the metric measurement always be listed on the patient's instructions and that the American standard measurement be given only when appropriate. Further, there are multiple ways of expressing the metric measurement of liquids; often "mL" and "cc" are used interchangeably. Adopting a standard practice of always typing "mL" is preferred, but the policies of each individual pharmacy will direct a pharmacy technician on what is expected.

Some prescriptions are for medical devices and supplies. Many pharmacies dispense blood glucose testing supplies to patients with diabetes and nebulizers to patients with breathing disorders, just to list a few of the many devices that pharmacies can be involved with dispensing. Prescriptions for devices often have very different requirements than prescriptions for drugs. Many times, a diagnosis or diagnosis code (also knows as an ICD or International Statistical Classification of Disease and Related Health Problems code) is required for billing insurance companies for medical devices and supplies. A technician may encounter these types of orders and must be familiar with seeing this extra information on such orders.

Examples of Prescriptions for Medical Devices and Supplies

Patient: Sally Sickly (DOB: 7/4/2004)
                                    Date Written: 2/24/2013

Nebulizer with Compressor
Sig: Direct Sally to inhale budesonide treatments
twice daily. Duration of need: Indefinite.
Diagnosis: Asthma, Chronic.
Disp#: 1. No Refills

Nebulizer Supplies: Tubing, Plastic Reusable
Nebulizer Cup, Filters
Sig: Use with Compressor and replace PRN
Disp#: one-month supply. Refills: PRN

Budesonide 0.5 mg/2 mL inhalation vials
Sig: Inhale one vialful through a nebulizer BID
Disp#: one-month supply. Refills: 6

                                    Dr. I. Respire
                                    NPI 8765234072

In the inpatient setting, orders are often documented digitally and are forwarded to the pharmacy through the institution's computer system. Medication orders in this setting have features that outpatient orders don't usually have; specific times for administration, a length of therapy or discontinuation date, and a lack of dispense quantity and refills can be used as distinguishing features for inpatient orders. Medications are usually delivered at specific times in a hospital or long-term care facility, so medication orders usually reflect the common delivery times for medications. For instance, 7 a.m., 1 p.m. and 7 p.m. could be common medication delivery times, so a three-times-per-day drug would likely be given at 7 a.m., 1 p.m. and 7 p.m. in a facility with this standard delivery schedule. Further, many drugs in the inpatient setting have a set duration for therapy, so orders must include the date to stop giving the drug. Finally, inpatient orders will not usually include a quantity to be dispensed because each dose will be administered individually to the patient based on a single medication order until the stop date specified on the medication order is reached.

Drug Enforcement Administration (DEA) Registration Numbers

The DEA is the federal agency that regulates controlled substances in the United States. In order for a pharmacy to dispense controlled substances, the pharmacy must be registered with the DEA. Neither pharmacists nor technicians register with the DEA; however, to have controlled substances in the pharmacies where they work, the pharmacy must be registered with the DEA. Prescribers who wish to write orders for controlled substances must also be registered with the DEA, as must many other facilities and individuals involved with the dispensing of controlled substances. Once registered, the DEA issues a unique number to the registrant. This number is structured in such a way that the final digit is a "check digit." This is done so that when a registrant lists his or her DEA number on a prescription or other form, the receiver of that prescription or form can verify that the number is at least a valid number and has not been written down incorrectly. To truly authenticate a DEA number, anyone who holds a DEA number can access the DEA's website (usdoj.gov/dea) to verify the authenticity of a DEA number. Although computers have made the need to know the formula to verify a DEA number's check digit virtually unnecessary, it is important that every pharmacist and technician know how to manually verify the check digit of a DEA number as the situation may arise where it must be done by hand.

Before looking at how to verify the check digit for a DEA number, one must first look at the anatomy of the number itself. A DEA number always begins with two letters. The first letter can be any of the following:

1. A, B or F for a physician, pharmacy or hospital
2. M for a mid-level prescriber/practitioner (e.g., a nurse practitioner or physician's assistant)
3. P or R for a drug wholesaler

The second letter is the first letter of the prescriber's last name or the facility name (e.g., Dr. Smith's DEA number could start FS and Smith's Pharmacy could start AS). One exception to this rule is when the DEA issues a number to a person or a facility and then the name of the person or facility changes; the DEA does not automatically update the DEA number due to a name change. Then, there is a series of seven digits, with the final digit being a check digit.

To find the check digit, do the following:

1. Add the first, third and fifth digits.
2. Add the second, fourth and sixth digits. Multiply this sum by two.
3. Add the sum from steps 1 and 2. The number farthest to the right is the check digit.
4. The check digit should be identical to the last digit (furthest right) in the DEA number.

EXAMPLE
Verifying a DEA Number

Verify DEA Number AP8043159 for Dr. Betty Pre-scriber.

Step 1: Add the first, third and fifth digits.

8 + 4 + 1 = 13

Step 2: Add the second, fourth and sixth digits. Multiply this sum by two.

0 + 3 + 5 = 8

8 x 2 = 16

Step 3: Add the sum from Steps 1 and 2. The number farthest to the right (in the "ones place") is the check digit.

13 + 16 = 29

9 is the check digit, which matches the last number in the DEA number.

Therefore, this DEA number is valid.

EXAMPLE
Verifying a DEA Number

A patient presents a prescription that looks suspicious. It is for morphine, and the patient has never been on morphine before. You call over your pharmacist who agrees that it looks a little out of the ordinary and asks you, her technician, to verify the DEA number listed on the prescription. You read that Dr. Nancy Jeffreys is the prescriber who signed the prescription. The DEA Number that was written in by the person who signed the prescription is: FR6561876.

You turn to your pharmacist and say, "I don't even have to grab a calculator! The second letter should be a 'J' not an 'R' – unless Dr. Jeffreys recently changed her name, this is likely a fake!"

National Provider Identifier (NPI)

Only prescribers who write for controlled substances and facilities that handle controlled substances need a DEA number; however, many insurance companies used to require that a DEA number be provided on many claims in order to identify the prescriber or pharmacy. This caused many problems with prescribers who didn't have a DEA number (and didn't necessarily need one) and so a national identifier system was adopted for not only physicians, but also all health care practitioners and health care facilities. Pharmacists, pharmacies, hospitals, nurses, respiratory therapists and any other provider can get an NPI. The NPI is issued by the National Plan & Provider Enumeration System (NPPES) and is free to all health care facilities and practitioners. Much like the DEA number, the NPI has a built-in check digit that most pharmacy computer systems will verify when an NPI is entered. To authenticate an NPI, NPPES has setup a website, nppes.cms.hhs.gov, where anyone may search for a provider to see if an NPI has been issued. Again, though, every pharmacist and technician needs to be familiar with how to validate an NPI's check digit manually in case the need ever arises.

Unlike a DEA number, there are no letters in an NPI. An NPI is a 10-digit number with the final number being the check digit. The NPI, or a similarly-named identifier, is used in many countries throughout the world for many different purposes (from banking to health care). So, prefixes are required in validation but are not usually listed as part of the NPI. With prefixes, the NPI is actually 15 digits. To validate an NPI, follow these steps:

1. Add the "hidden" prefix of 80840 to the NPI.
   a. 80 is the prefix for health care
   b. 840 is the second prefix identifying this as a number from the United States
2. Starting with the leftmost number as position one, double the numbers in positions 2, 4, 6, 8, 10, 12 and 14 and record your results. If this doubling results in a number 10 or greater, record each digit of the sum separately (e.g., 14 would be recorded as 1 and 4).
3. Add all of the digits obtained from Step 2 to the numbers in positions 1, 3, 5, 7, 9, 11 and 13 from the NPI number in question.
4. Subtract the sum obtained in Step 3 from the next highest number ending in 0 (if the sum from step 3 is 0, then record 0). This is the check digit and should be in the rightmost position of the NPI. For example, if the sum from step 3 is 22, the next highest number ending in 0 is 30. Therefore, 30 - 22 = 8, which should match the number furthest to the right in the NPI number.

EXAMPLE
Validating an NPI Number

Validate the NPI 1124049176.

Position	1	2	3	4	5	6	7	8	9	10	11	12	13	14	Check
NPI	8	0	8	4	0	1	1	2	4	0	4	9	1	7	6
x2		0		8		2		4		0		1,8		1,4	
Add	8+0+8+8+0+2+1+4+4+0+4+(1+8)+1+(1+4) = 54														
Subtract	60 – 54 =														6
Check?															OK

EXAMPLE
Validating an NPI Number

Validate the NPI 1023262005.

Position	1	2	3	4	5	6	7	8	9	10	11	12	13	14	Check
NPI	8	0	8	4	0	1	0	2	3	2	6	2	0	0	5
x2		0		8		2		4		4		4		0	
Add	8+0+8+8+0+2+0+4+3+4+6+4+0+0 = 47														
Subtract	50 – 47 =														3
Check?															NO

References

1. Traupman, John C. The Bantam New College Latin & English Dictionary. New York, NY: Bantam Books, 1995.

Chapter 5
PRACTICE PROBLEMS

Convert between the abbreviation and the English meaning by filling in the missing side of each equation:

1. QAM = ?

2. QID = ?

3. Twice weekly = ?

4. After a meal = ?

5. ODT = ?

6. D5NS = ?

7. At bedtime = ?

8. †̄†̄†̄ = ?

9. †̄ / †̄†̄ SL AC and QHS PRN Abdominal Pain = ?

10. As needed for pain = ?

11. Unwrap and insert one suppository rectally every four to six hours as needed for nausea and vomiting = ?

12. BID = ?

13. TID = ?

14. Extended release = ?

15. IVPB = ?

Convert between Roman numerals and Arabic numerals by filling in the missing side of the equation:

16. II = ?

17. XI = ?

18. MCM = ?

19. DLVII = ?

20. MCMXCVIII = ?

21. 725 = ?

22. 1,492 = ?

23. 25 = ?

24. CMXXXIV = ?

25. 5,399 = ?

26. XXXVIII = ?

27. XLIV = ?

Yes or No: Are the following DEA numbers valid for the prescriber or facility?

28. Dr. Andrew Smith: FS7826451

29. Nurse Practitioner John Appleseed: AJ7462118

30. Walt's Downtown Pharmacy: AW8053148

31. Send-It-Back Wholesaler: RW9650090

Yes or No: Are the following NPIs valid?

32. 1234567893

33. 8764535465

34. 6756694527

35. 7777777777

Interpret the following orders by answering the questions following each prescription example.

```
┌─────────────────────────────────────────────────────┐
│  Patient: Askin Y. Me                                 │
│  DOB: 04/15/2004                                      │
│                                                       │
│            Amoxicillin 250 mg/5 mL                    │
│          Sig: 2 teaspoonfuls BID x21d                 │
│              Give QS / No Refills                     │
│                                                       │
│                              Dr. A.B. Overkill        │
│                    Date Written: 3 March 2013         │
└─────────────────────────────────────────────────────┘
```

36. What action verb and route of administration would be appropriate for the label for this medication?

37. Write out this prescription as it would be read.

```
┌─────────────────────────────────────────────────────┐
│  Patient: Lotsov Payne                                │
│  DOB: 7/4/1972                                        │
│                                                       │
│   Hydrocodone / APAP 7.5 mg / 750 mg Tablets          │
│            Sig: Ť/ŤŤ Q4/6H P/P                        │
│  Quantity: 360 (three hundred sixty) / Refills: 3 (three) │
│                                                       │
│                          Dr. May B. Aye, D.O.         │
│                          DEA FA7356923                │
│                    Date Written: 3/14/2013            │
└─────────────────────────────────────────────────────┘
```

38. What is the most appropriate action verb and route of administration for the prescription label for this medication?

39. How would the sig read when typed out on the patient's label?

```
Patient: Ms. Rhino, Rhea
D.O.B.: 7/7/1977

                Fluticasone
          †/†† IEN up to BID PRN
        Q.S. 90-day supply / Ref: PRN

                        Flo Aqua, N.P.
                   NPI: 7777777789
              Date Written: 1/2/2013
```

40.   How would the sig read when typed out on the patient's label?

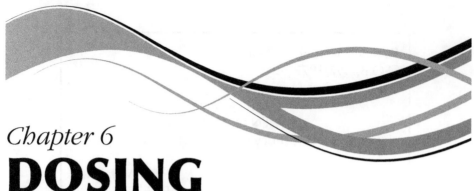

Chapter 6

DOSING REGIMENS AND DOSAGE CALCULATIONS

By Karen Woods Miron, R.Ph.

Learning Objectives

Upon completion of this chapter, the technician should be able to:
- learn different methods of calculating doses for patients.
- calculate appropriate doses for patients based on weight and body surface area.
- determine body surface area (BSA) using nomograms.
- determine the number of days supply of medications using dosing regimens.

Introduction

Pharmacy professionals are frequently involved in calculating a patient's dose or interpreting a dosing regimen as prescribed by a health care provider. We are often asked to convert dosing based on age, weight, kidney function or other factors. When preparing prescription orders, it is often necessary to determine the quantity of medication to be dispensed for the course of therapy or duration of treatment. It is important for pharmacy technicians to be able to perform these types of calculations so they can assist in the dispensing process and double check the pharmacist's calculations to minimize medication errors.

Dosing Regimens

A **dosing regimen** is the schedule of medication administration. A dosing regimen usually includes the name of the drug, the quantity or concentration of the drug and its frequency or schedule of administration. Pharmacy professionals frequently determine the amount or number of units of a medication to be dispensed from a dosage regimen and a prescribed number of days for therapy. Examples of dosing regimens follow.

lorazepam 1 mg b.i.d. prn

cefixime suspension 100 mg/5 mL give 200 mg every 12 hr for 10 days

ifosfamide 1.2 g/m² IV for 5 days every 3 weeks

Calculating the amount of drug product to dispense or day's supply from a dosage regimen is a daily function for pharmacy professionals. It is done to ensure the appropriate amount of medication is dispensed to the patient, is utilized when billing third party payors and is performed when preparing intravenous medications. Most of the calculations can be done by using simple mathematical principles such as multiplication, division and proportions.

Calculating the Amount of Medication to Dispense

The most common calculations in the pharmacy are determining the amount of medication needed to fill a prescription and determining a month's supply.

$$\text{Total doses needed} = \frac{\text{dose}}{\text{day}} \times \text{days supply}$$

$$\text{Days supply} = \frac{\text{total doses needed}}{\text{dose/day}}$$

EXAMPLE
Determining Total Doses Needed

A patient needs Erythromycin, one 500 mg tablet t.i.d. for 10 days. Determine amount of tablets to dispense.

Step 1: Insert known amounts into equation.

$$\text{Number of doses} = \frac{3 \text{ tablets}}{\text{day}} \times 10 \text{ days}$$

Step 2: Solve for number of doses.

$$\text{Number of doses} = \frac{3 \text{ tablets}}{\text{day}} \times 10 \text{ days}$$

Number of doses = 3 tablets x 10

Number of doses = 30 tablets

EXAMPLE
Determining Quantity to Dispense for Month's Supply

A prescription is written for megestrol 40 mg 4 times daily. Your pharmacy stocks 20 mg tablets. Determine the quantity of tablets to dispense for a 30-day supply.

Step 1: Calculate the dose/day.

40 mg = 2 tablets of 20 mg

$$2 \text{ tablets} \times \frac{4 \text{ doses}}{\text{day}} = 8 \text{ tablets/day}$$

Step 2: Multiply tablets/day by number of days needed.

$$\text{Total doses needed} = \frac{\text{dose}}{\text{day}} \times \text{days supply}$$

Total number of doses to dispense =

$$\frac{8 \text{ tablets}}{\text{day}} \times 30 \text{ days}$$

Total number of doses to dispense = 8 x 30 tablets = 240 tablets

Often, the calculation of number of doses, total amount of drug and size of dose are more complicated than multiplying tablets. Dosage calculations can always be solved by knowing the relationship of number of doses, total amount of drug and size of dose. By knowing any two pieces of information, you can always solve for the third.

$$\text{number of doses} = \frac{\text{total amount of drug}}{\text{size of dose}}$$

total amount of drug = number of doses x size of dose

$$\text{size of doses} = \frac{\text{total amount of drug}}{\text{number of doses}}$$

EXAMPLE
Determining Days Supply

You have a 10 mL vial of insulin that has 100 units/mL. Your patient injects 35 units twice daily. How many days will one vial of 10 mL last?

Step 1: Determine the total number of units in one vial.

$$\text{units/vial} = \frac{100 \text{ units}}{\text{mL}} \times \frac{10 \text{ mL}}{\text{vial}}$$

$$\text{units/vial} = \frac{100 \text{ units} \times 10}{\text{vial}}$$

$$\text{units/vial} = 1{,}000 \text{ units}$$

Step 2: Determine the number of doses in one vial.

$$\text{number of doses} = \frac{\text{total amount of drug}}{\text{size of dose}}$$

$$\text{Number of doses} = \frac{1{,}000 \text{ units}}{35 \text{ units}}$$

Number of doses = 28.57 doses
(Rounded to whole doses = 28)

Step 3: Determine the days supply:

$$\text{Days supply} = \frac{\text{Total number of doses}}{\text{dose/day}}$$

$$\text{Days supply} = \frac{28 \text{ doses}}{2 \text{ doses/day}}$$

Days supply = 14 days

Tip: The total amount of drug needed and the size of dose available must be converted to the same units before solving any equation. In dosing by weight, it is extremely important to note if the weight is listed in pounds or kilograms. There are 2.2 pounds in a kilogram, so if the units are not converted, a significant error would occur.

Milligrams per Kilogram per Day Method

This method of calculating doses can apply to adults and children, is widely accepted in pharmacy practice and, therefore, is typically used to calculate dosages. Many manufacturers reference dosage recommendations in package inserts utilizing this method. Following are the formulas illustrating this method.

dose per unit of weight (mg/kg) x weight of patient (kg) = dose (mg)

dose per kg per day (mg/kg/day) x weight of patient (kg) = dose per day (mg/day)

EXAMPLE
Determining the Size of a Patient's Dose Based on Weight

If prednisone is needed at 1 mg/kg/day in three divided doses for a child weighing 44 pounds, what would his daily dose be? What would each dose be?

Step 1: Convert the patient's weight in pounds (44) to kilograms. (Remember that 2.2 lb equals 1 kg.)

44 lb ÷ 2.2 lb/kg = patient's weight in kilograms

$$44 \, \cancel{lb} \times \frac{kg}{2.2 \, \cancel{lb}} = \text{patient's weight in kilograms}$$

$$\frac{44}{2.2} = 20 \text{ kg}$$

Therefore, a 44 lb patient weighs 20 kg.

Step 2: Determine the total amount of drug/day required using multiplication.

Since 1 mg/kg/day has been prescribed, calculate the total amount of prednisone required per day by using simple multiplication.

1 mg/kg/day x 20 kg = total amount of drug required

1 mg/$\cancel{kg}$/day x 20 $\cancel{kg}$ = total amount of drug required

1 mg/day x 20 = 20 mg/day

Therefore, the total amount of prednisone required is 20 mg/day.

Step 3: Use the following formula to solve for the unknown, the size of a single dose. (The wording "in three divided doses" means the child would get three equal doses per day to equal a total of 1mg/kg/day)

$$\text{size of dose} = \frac{\text{total amount of drug}}{\text{number of doses}}$$

$$\text{size of dose} = \frac{20 \text{ mg}}{3 \text{ doses}}$$

$$\text{size of dose} = 6.67 \text{ mg}$$

Therefore, the size of each prednisone dose is 6.67 mg.

EXAMPLE

Determining the Number of Doses Needed by a Patient

The doctor from the previous example wants the patient to take the prednisone for seven days before returning to the doctor's office for further evaluation. Using information from the previous example, determine how many doses the patient will need.

Step 1: Find total amount needed for seven days.

Since the total amount of prednisone was only calculated for one day in the previous example, total amount needed for seven days must be found by multiplying the amount of medication per day by seven days.

$$\frac{20 \text{ mg}}{\text{day}} \text{ \# 7 days total amount of drug needed}$$

$$\frac{20 \text{ mg}}{\text{day}} \text{ \# 7 } \cancel{\text{days}} = \text{total amount of drug}$$

20 mg x 7 = 140 mg

Therefore, 140 mg of prednisone are needed to treat a patient for seven days.

Step 2: Insert the known quantities into the equation and solve for number of doses.

$$\text{number of doses} = \frac{\text{total amount of drug}}{\text{size of dose}}$$

$$\text{number of doses} = 140 \text{ mg} \div \frac{6.67 \text{ mg}}{\text{doses}}$$

$$\text{number of doses} = 140 \text{ \sout{mg}} \div \frac{\text{doses}}{6.67 \text{ \sout{mg}}}$$

$$\text{number of doses} = \frac{140 \text{ doses}}{6.67}$$

number of doses = 20.995 rounded to 21 doses

Therefore, the number of prednisone doses needed for seven days of treatment is 21 doses.

This problem could have also been easily solved by using simple logic and multiplication as demonstrated in the following equation.

$$\frac{3 \text{ doses}}{\text{day}} \times 7 \text{ days} = \text{total number of doses}$$

$$\frac{3 \text{ doses}}{\text{\sout{day}}} \times 7 \text{ \sout{days}} = \text{total number of doses}$$

3 doses x 7 = 21 doses

Therefore, the number of prednisone doses needed for seven days of treatment is 21 doses, regardless of the method used.

EXAMPLE
Determining Total Amount of Drug Required by a Patient

How much prednisone 5 mg/mL solution do you need to dispense in order to give the child enough for 7 days?

Step 1: Calculate amount to dispense using the equation:

total amount of drug =
number of doses x size of dose

$$\text{total amount of drug} = 21 \text{ doses} \times \frac{1.32 \text{ mL}}{\text{dose}}$$

$$\text{total amount of drug} = 21 \text{ \sout{doses}} \times \frac{1.32 \text{ mL}}{\text{\sout{dose}}}$$

total amount of drug = 27.72 mL

Therefore, you would dispense 28 mL of prednisone 5 mg/mL solution.

EXAMPLE
Determining a Dose Based on Weight

A physician orders 35 mcg/kg/day of digoxin for a patient in your pharmacy. The pharmacist is instructed to adjust the dose monthly based on the child's weight. The mother reports to you that the baby has gained weight and is now at 13 pounds 6 ounces. Determine the baby's daily dose.

Step 1: Calculate the baby's weight in pounds. First, convert ounces to pounds.

1 lb = 16 oz

$$6 \text{ oz} \times \frac{1 \text{ lb}}{16 \text{ oz}} = 0.375 \text{ lb}$$

Then, add the pounds together.

13 lbs + 0.375 lbs = 13.375 lbs

Step 2: Convert pounds to kilograms

1 kilogram = 2.2 pounds

$$\text{Weight in kg} = 13.375 \text{ lb} \div \frac{2.2 \text{ lb}}{\text{kg}} =$$

$$13.375 \text{ \sout{lb}} \times \frac{1 \text{ kg}}{2.2 \text{ \sout{lb}}} = \frac{13.375 \text{ kg}}{2.2}$$

Weight in kg = 6.079 kg rounded to 6.1 kg

Step 3: Solve for daily dose (Z).

$$Z = 35 \text{ mcg/kg/day} \times 6.1 \text{ kg}$$

$$Z = \frac{35 \text{ mcg}}{\cancel{\text{kg}}\text{/day}} \times 6.1 \cancel{\text{kg}}$$

$$Z = \frac{35 \text{ mcg} \times 6.1}{\text{day}}$$

$$Z = 213.5 \text{ mcg/day}$$

Children's Dosages

Doses listed in medical references are typically based on the amount of medication needed to treat the average sized adult (150 lb or 68 kg). When a drug is commonly used for children, the pediatric dose will be listed and should be consulted. However, pediatric doses are not always listed. If the adult dose is the only known dose, calculations based on weight may be performed. A preferred method is calculating the dose based on Body Surface Area (BSA) or nomogram. The formula used depends on what information is available.

Body Surface Area or Nomogram Method

The nomogram method of calculating dosages is accurate because it is based upon the patient's size. It takes into consideration the person's body surface area (BSA) in meters squared (m^2), with 1.73 m^2 being the surface area of the average adult. The BSA for a child is determined from a nomogram that calculates BSA from the weight (mass) and height of the child. BSA is often used to calculate doses for patients receiving chemotherapy, both adults and children. Following is the pediatric formula for calculating dosage using BSA.

$$\text{child's dose} = \frac{\text{child's BSA}(m^2)}{1.73 \text{ m}^2} \times \text{adult dose}$$

Before using this formula, however, you must determine the BSA. To determine BSA, use the nomograms in Figures 1 and 2. Please note that there is a nomogram for children and a different nomogram for adults. To solve for BSA, follow these five steps:

1. Use the appropriate nomogram for an adult or child.
2. Find the patient's weight in pounds or kilograms on the right-hand side of the nomogram and place a dot next to the weight.
3. Find the patient's height in inches or centimeters on the left-hand side of the nomogram and place a dot on the height.
4. Draw a straight line connecting these two points.
5. Read the patient's BSA, located on the center vertical line at the intersection where the line in Step 4 intersects the center line.

Figure 1: Nomogram for Children

Determination of body surface from height and mass[1]

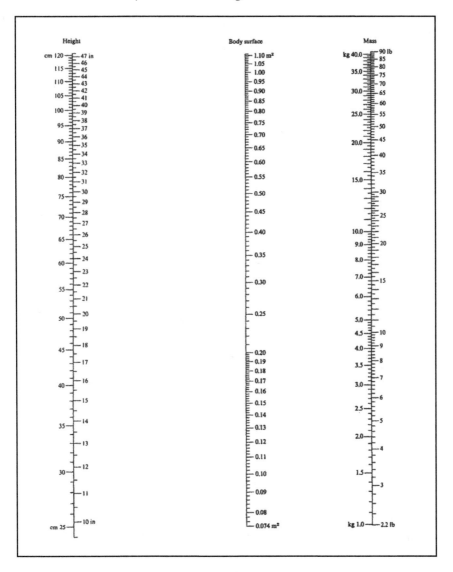

[1]From the formula of Du Bois and Du Bois, Arch Intern Med, 17, 863 (1916): S = $M^{0.425}$ x $H^{0.725}$ x 71.84, or log S = log M x 0.425 + log H x 0.725 + 1.8564 (S = body surface in cm^2, M = mass in kg, H = height in cm).

Source: C. Lenter, Ed., Geigy Scientific Tables, 8th edition, Vol. 1 Basel: Ciba-Geigy; 1981: 226-227.

Figure 2: Nomogram for Adults

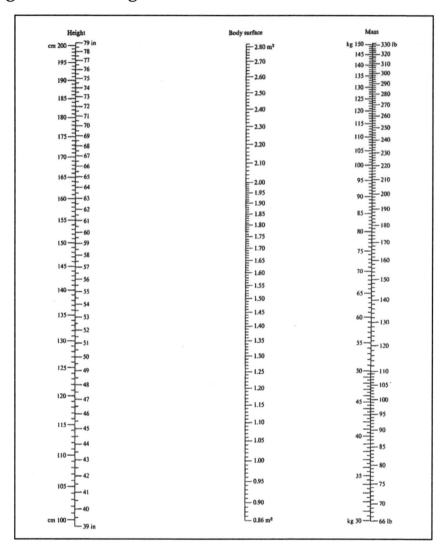

[1]From the formula of Du Bois and Du Bois, Arch Intern Med, 17, 863 (1916): S = $M^{0.425}$ x $H^{0.725}$ x 71.84, or log S = log M x 0.425 + log H x 0.725 + 1.8564 (S = body surface in cm^2, M = mass in kg, H = height in cm).

Source: C. Lenter, Ed., Geigy Scientific Tables, 8th edition, Vol. 1
Basel: Ciba-Geigy; 1981: 226-227.

EXAMPLE
Determining BSA for a Child

What is the BSA for a child who is 50 cm tall and weighs 20 lb?

Step 1: Be sure you are using the child nomogram.

Step 2: Place dots on the 50-cm mark (left column) and on the 20-lb mark (right column).

Step 3: Connect the dots with a straight line.

Step 4: Locate the point at which the line crosses the body surface area column (middle column).

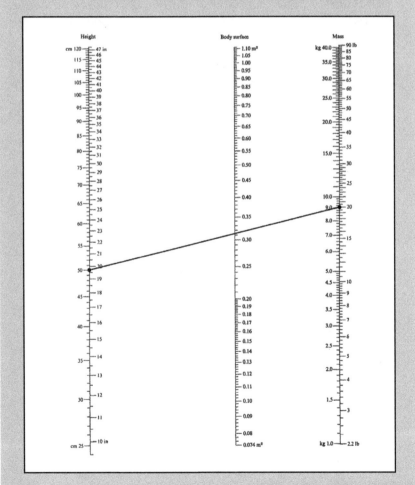

Therefore, the BSA for this child is 0.315 m^2.

EXAMPLE
Determining BSA for Adults

What is the BSA for an adult who is 5′ 9″ tall and weighs 84 kg?

Step 1: Be sure you are using the adult nomogram.

Step 2: Convert height to inches.

5′ 9″ = 69″

Step 3: Place dots on the 69-in mark (left column) and on the 84-kg mark (right column).

Step 4: Connect the dots with a straight line.

Step 5: Locate the point at which the line crosses the body surface area column (middle column).

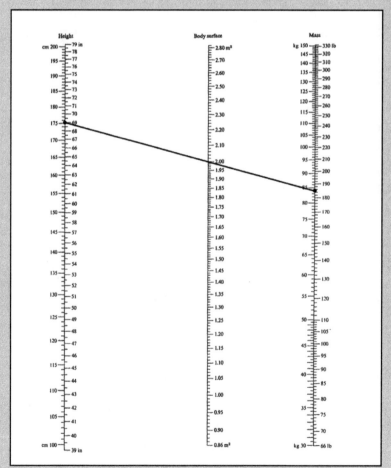

Therefore, the BSA for this adult is 2 m².

Tip: Dosage formulas that involve a patient's size (weight or body surface area) are more accurate than formulas that deal with age.

EXAMPLE
Calculating Dose Based on BSA

If the adult dose for micafungin is 150 mg I.V. daily, using the information from the previous example (BSA = 0.315 m²), what is the appropriate dose for a child who is 50 cm tall and weighs 20 lb?

Step 1: Insert the known amounts into the equation and complete.

$$\text{child's dose} = \frac{\text{child's BSA}(m^2)}{1.73 \ m^2} \times \text{adult dose}$$

$$\text{child's dose} = \frac{0.315 \ m^2}{1.73 \ m^2} \times 150 \ mg$$

$$\text{child's dose} = \frac{0.315 \ \cancel{m^2}}{1.73 \ \cancel{m^2}} \times 150 \ mg$$

$$\text{child's dose} = \frac{0.315 \times 150 \ mg}{1.73}$$

$$\text{child's dose} = \frac{47.25 \ mg}{1.73}$$

$$\text{child's dose} = 27.312 \ mg$$

Therefore, the child's dose should be 27.312 mg (rounded to 27 mg).

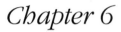

Chapter 6
PRACTICE PROBLEMS

1. If a patient weighs 65 kg and the usual preoperative dose of midazolam is 0.08 mg/kg, what would the dose for this patient be?

2. If chloral hydrate is dosed at 25 mg/kg/day as a sedative for children, what is the dose for a 40 lb child?

3. If a dose of a medication is 75 mg/kg/day in four divided doses, what is the dose for a 220 lb patient?

4. The doctor orders glucagon 25 mcg/kg for an infant who is severely hypoglycemic. If the infant weighs 12 pounds, what would the dose of glucagon be?

5. If the dose of a medication is 35 mg/kg/day in four divided doses, what is the dose for a 125 lb patient?

6. If the dose of a medication is 18 mg/kg/day in three divided doses, what is the dose for a 275 lb patient?

7. Determine the number of grams of medication to dispense in the following dosing regimen: Ibuprofen 800 mg – take one tablet t.i.d. for 5 days

8. If the physician prescribes Darvocet N-100 po 1 to 2 tablets every 4-6 hours PRN for 3 days, what is the maximum number of tablets that should be dispensed?

Use the following scenario to solve problems 9 through 12:

A physician prescribes phenytoin 6 mg/kg/day divided into three daily doses for a 163-pound female patient to control convulsions. The physician is investigating using 150 mg phenytoin capsules compounded by the pharmacy, instead of the commercially-available options, in order to reduce the number of capsules the patient must take each day.

9. How much phenytoin should be administered for each dose?

10. If the doctor prescribed the phenytoin for a total of 5 days, how many milligrams of medication should be dispensed?

11. The pharmacy is unable to compound 150 mg capsules and must order the commercially-available 50 mg chewable tablets. How many tablets would be dispensed for 10 days of therapy?

12. The patient continues to experience convulsions, so the physician increases the daily dose to 8 mg/kg/day. The pharmacy is able to once-again compound the 150 mg capsules. How many 150 mg capsules will the patient take each day?

Use the following scenario to solve problems 13 and 14:

A geriatric patient who has difficulty swallowing large tablets presents a prescription for Erythromycin 400 mg/5 mL with directions to take 500 mg every 12 hours for 10 days.

13. Determine the amount of suspension needed to make one 500 mg dose.

14. Determine the volume of medication to be dispensed for the full course of therapy.

Use the following scenario to solve problems 15 and 16:

A 14-month-old child weighs 11 kg and is 79 cm tall.

15. What is the child's BSA? See the Nomogram for Children (Figure 1).

16. What would the medication dose for this child be if the medication is normally dosed as 12 mg/m^2 ?

Use the following scenario to solve problems 17 and 18:

A 36-year-old female patient weighs 161 pounds and is 5 feet 7 inches tall.

17. What is the patient's BSA? See Nomogram for Adults (Figure 2).

18. If the patient were to take medication normally dosed at 30 mg/m^2, what would her dose be?

Use the following scenario to solve problems 19 and 20:

Theophyllin 100 mg tablets are prescribed for the treatment of asthma and have a recommended dose of 3 mg/kg of body weight every eight hours. The patient weighs 219 pounds, and the doctor would like the patient to take the medication for 14 days before returning to the office for further evaluation.

19. What dose is required for this patient?

20. How many 100 mg tablets should be dispensed to this patient to complete the 14-day regimen?

Patient: N.O. Cena	
DOB: 5/5/1955	
24-hour Total Parenteral (IV) Nutrition (TPN)	

Ingredient / Nutrient	Amount to Add
Dextrose 5%	850 mL
Amino Acids with Electrolytes 8.5%	500 mL
Lipids 10%	500 mL
Calcium Gluconate 10%	1 g
Potassium Chloride 2 mEq/mL	40 mEq
MVI	10 mL
Trace Elements	1 mL
Insulin Regular 100 units/mL	100 units

Dr. I.V. Sticker
Date Written: 2/18/2013

21. How much potassium chloride will be added to this TPN bag?

22. How much calcium gluconate solution will be added to this TPN bag?

Patient: Mr. Albert Lerjick
D.O.B.: 2/10/1950

Prednisone 10 mg Tablets
Sig: 6 tabs x3d, 5 tabs x3d, 4 tabs x2d, ††† x3d,
†† x2d, † x4d, 1/2-Tab x3d
Disp: Q.S. Ref: 2

Dr. Stuff E. Knows
NPI: 8620090078

23. How many 10 mg tablets must be dispensed to fill this prescription?

24. This patient will not be able to split these tablets in half due to significant arthritis of the hands, so your pharmacist asks you to dispense 5 mg tablets for the whole prescription instead. How many tablets must be given?

25. How many days will a fill of this prescription last?

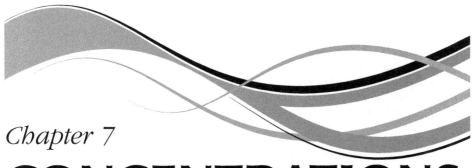

Chapter 7

CONCENTRATIONS AND DILUTIONS

By Derek J. Quinn, Pharm.D.

Learning Objectives

Upon completion of this chapter, the technician should be able to:
- define concentration and be familiar with how concentrations are commonly expressed.
- convert between knowing the concentration of a mixture and writing a recipe for a mixture.
- set up equal fractions (also known as cross-multiplication) to solve concentration and dilution problems.
- define dilution and be familiar with how diluting a mixture affects its concentration.
- determine the recipe needed to dilute a solution.
- either solve the algebraic equation or use the visual alligation method to determine the recipe for a mixture made by compounding two mixtures together.
- apply the skills discussed in this chapter to manipulate a concentration-based medication order.

Introduction

Any time a pharmacist or pharmacy technician mixes two different liquids or solids together, a mixture with a measurable concentration is formed. Knowing how to convert back and forth between determining the concentration of a particular mixture and determining the recipe for a mixture is not only a handy tool but also an important task regularly performed by pharmacy technicians. In fact, considering how many liquids, creams, ointments, gels and other mixtures are dispensed each day (each of them having a concentration value), understanding how to interpret a concentration value, or determine a recipe from a concentration value, is a truly invaluable skill for a pharmacy technician. Further, assisting a pharmacist who is tasked with mixture creation provides a professional opportunity for a pharmacy technician.

Terms

When talking about mixtures, it is important to have a few terms clearly defined as they are not always interchangeable. The following definitions provide a scientific understanding, with a practical example, of the terms commonly referred to when talking about mixtures.

Diluent: An "inert substance added to source material to thin it to the potency [or concentration] desired." (e.g., water)

Heterogeneous: "Composed of different substances or different phases [solid/liquid/gas] of the same substance." A mixture where different substances can be clearly seen within the mixture. (e.g., chocolate chip cookies)

Homogeneous: Composed of a "uniform composition or structure." A mixture that appears the same throughout. (e.g., chocolate milk)

Mixture: "A composition of two or more substances that are not chemically combined with each other and are capable of being separated." (e.g., chocolate chip cookies)

Solute: "A substance that is dissolved in another substance (a solvent), forming a solution." (e.g., chocolate syrup is the solute, milk is the solvent, chocolate milk is the mixture)

Solution: "A mixture in which particles of one or more substances (the solute) are distributed uniformly throughout another substance (the solvent), so that the mixture is homogeneous at the molecular or ionic level. The particles in a solution are smaller than those in ... a suspension." (e.g., chocolate milk)

Solvent: "A substance that can dissolve another substance, or in which another substance is dissolved, forming a solution." (e.g., milk before the chocolate is added)

Suspension: "A mixture in which small particles of a substance are dispersed throughout a ... liquid. If a suspension is left undisturbed, the particles are likely to settle to the bottom. The particles in a suspension are larger than those in ... a solution." (e.g., amoxicillin suspension)

Concentration

A concentration can be measured whenever two or more substances are mixed together; since pharmacists rarely work with gases, the types of mixtures being made or used in pharmacies involve solids mixed with solids, liquids mixed with liquids, or solids mixed with liquids. The concentration of any mixture in pharmacy is expressed by taking the amount of drug in the mixture and dividing that by the total volume or weight of the mixture. Thus, depending on if solids or liquids are being mixed, the units on the concentration must change as indicated below:

Solid + Solid = %w/w (percent weight/weight)
   This is the weight in grams (g) of drug present in one hundred grams (100 g) of the mixture. Since both the drug and the total mixture are

weighed in grams, the units (g/g) cancel out and the concentration is expressed as a percentage (%).

For example, betamethasone dipropionate 0.05% cream contains 0.05 g of betamethasone dipropionate for every 100 g of cream dispensed (the other 99.05 g is the cream base).

Liquid + Liquid = %v/v (percent volume/volume)

This is the volume in milliliters (mL) of drug present in one hundred milliliters (100 mL) of the mixture. Since the volume of both the drug and the total mixture are being compared (and are measured in milliliters), the units (mL/mL) cancel out and the concentration is expressed as a percentage (%).

For example, hydrogen peroxide 3% solution contains 3 mL of hydrogen peroxide for every 100 mL dispensed (the other 97 mL is a solvent).

Solid + Liquid = %w/v (percent weight/volume)

This is the weight in grams (g) of drug present in one hundred milliliters (100 mL) of the mixture. Since the weight of the drug and the volume of the solution are measured in different units (weight is measured in grams (g) and volume is measured in milliliters (mL)), the units do not cancel and must both be present when reporting the concentration. Note that many solid drugs are added in very small quantities compared to the volume of the final product; therefore, concentration is commonly expressed as milligrams/milliliter (mg/mL). Further note that sometimes the units are not reported and the concentration is listed as simply a percentage (e.g., 0.9% (normal) saline, 5% dextrose in water); in this case, it must be assumed that the units of g/mL apply.

For example, oxybutinin 0.1 g/100 mL (another way to express this concentration is 1 mg/1 mL) solution contains 0.1 g (100 mg) of oxybutinin powder in every 100 mL of liquid dispensed.

Using this information, a pharmacy technician can find the final concentration of a compound based on the recipe for the compound or can write a recipe for a product based on the expressed concentration.

Another way of expressing concentration that is often used for very small amounts of a substance in a very large space is the "parts per" notation. For example, a study found the air to contain chlorofluorocarbons (CFC) at a concentration of 300 ppb (300 parts per billion). Using this CFC example, if you had a balloon that held one billion one-inch by one-inch cubes, then three hundred of those cubes would be filled with CFC and the rest would be filled with air. Parts per million (ppm) and parts per billion (ppb) are the most common units for such low concentrations. This notation is rarely used in pharmacy practice; however, it is used occasionally in scientific (including pharmaceutical) research and continuing education articles. Therefore, a pharmacy technician is expected to understand the use of the "parts per" notation as a way of expressing a concentration.

EXAMPLE
Using a Proportion to Solve for an Unknown Concentration

A patient has a prescription from her dermatologist ordering 6% salicylic acid powder (solid) in 120 g desoximetasone ointment (solid) to treat psoriasis. The pharmacist asks you to determine how much salicylic acid she will need to add to reach 6%.

Step 1: Convert the percentage to a fraction.

Express 6% w/w as how many grams of salicylic acid would be in 100 g of the mixture:

$$6\%\frac{w}{w} = \frac{6\text{ g salicylic acid}}{100\text{ g mixture}}$$

Step 2: Multiply the total weight of the mixture with the concentration fraction in Step 1.

$$\frac{120\text{ g mixture}}{1} \times \frac{6\text{ g salicylic acid}}{100\text{ g mixture}} =$$

$$\frac{720\text{ g salicylic acid}}{100} = 7.2\text{ g salicylic acid}$$

You present your calculation to your pharmacist and tell her that 7.2 g of salicylic acid powder should be added to 120 g of desoximetasone to make the compound a 6% salicylic acid mixture, and she agrees.

Concentration Conversions

A pharmacy technician must also be able to convert between concentrations using equal fractions (also known as cross-multiplication). Among other functions, this is useful when working backwards to check if a compound has been prepared correctly. First, we will look at how a recipe can be derived from knowing the concentration and the final volume.

EXAMPLE
Deriving a Recipe From Concentration and Volume

Your pharmacist needs to check your work after he asks you to help prepare a compound. The prescription calls for 480 mL of 5% hydrocortisone (solid) in diphenhydramine solution (liquid) to be compounded as a rinse to treat mouth sores. You do the calculations to determine how much hydrocortisone to add and begin preparing the compound. After weighing the hydrocortisone and properly mixing it into the diphenhydramine, you present your recipe, the ingredient stock bottles, final compound and a record from the scale stating that you weighed out 24 g of hydrocortisone.

The pharmacist checks your work by first noting that the final compound is 480 mL. Then, he reads your recipe, which reads as follows:

Mix 24 g of hydrocortisone powder and Q.S. Diphenhydramine liquid through a mortar to 480 mL.

Then, he begins calculating:

Step 1: Set up equal fractions comparing the amount of drug and the unknown amount that is in the volume of the final compound.

$$\frac{5 \text{ g hydrocortisone}}{100 \text{ mL mixture}} = \frac{Z \text{ g hydrocortisone}}{480 \text{ mL mixture}}$$

Step 2: Cross multiply to solve for the unknown (Z).

100 mL mixture x Z g hydrocortisone =
5 g hydrocortisone x 480 mL mixture

Divide both sides by 100 mL to isolate Z.

$$\frac{\cancel{100 \text{ mL mixture}} \times Z \text{ g hydrocortisone}}{\cancel{100 \text{ mL mixture}}} =$$

$$\frac{5 \text{ g hydrocortisone} \times 480 \cancel{\text{ mL mixture}}}{100 \cancel{\text{ mL mixture}}}$$

$$Z \text{ g hydrocortisone} = \frac{2,400 \text{ g hydrocortisone}}{100}$$

$$Z \text{ g hydrocortisone} = 24 \text{ g hydrocortisone}$$

Your work checks out and the compound is ready for dispensing.

Pharmacy technicians also can use a recipe for a product to determine its final concentration.

EXAMPLE
Determining Final Concentration From a Recipe

A prescription comes to the pharmacy calling for 20 g hydrocortisone powder (solid) to be added to 120 g of diphenhydramine cream to treat an itchy red rash. You know that you'll need to put the concentration of hydrocortisone on the label and set out to determine that concentration.

Step 1: Set up equal fractions comparing the recipe to the unknown amount of drug that would be in 100 g of the mixture.

$$\frac{20 \text{ g hydrocortisone}}{120 \text{ g mixture}} = \frac{Z \text{ g hydrocortisone}}{100 \text{ g mixture}}$$

Step 2: Isolate the unknown (Z) to solve.

$$\frac{100 \text{ g mixture}}{1} \times \frac{20 \text{ g hydrocortisone}}{120 \text{ g mixture}} =$$

$$\frac{Z \text{ g hydrocortisone}}{100 \text{ g mixture}} \times \frac{100 \text{ g mixture}}{1}$$

$$\frac{2,000 \text{ g hydrocortisone}}{120} = Z \text{ g hydrocortisone}$$

16.7 g hydrocortisone = Z g hydrocortisone

You determine that since there would be 16.7 g in 100 g of the final product, that the final product is 16.7%

hydrocortisone. Your pharmacist agrees and asks you to type the label to dispense this compound.

Each of these examples involved only one ingredient being mixed into a base. Many compounds and nearly all commercially-available products include multiple ingredients. When compounding, the concentration of each ingredient may need to be calculated, or a recipe may need to be written, from the concentrations provided for each ingredient. In the practice problems, multiple ingredient scenarios will be presented; the same steps must be followed and repeated for each ingredient.

Dilutions

In many cases, it is more economical for a pharmacy to purchase highly concentrated (lots of drug in very little volume or weight) mixtures and then dilute the stock mixture by adding a diluent (often the solvent used to prepare the concentrated mixture). During a dilution, the amount of drug in the mixture does not change; but, the volume in which it is dissolved does change. Since concentration is always expressed as a fraction, thinking about how a dilution changes the fraction helps clarify what is happening during a dilution. When a dilution is performed, the numerator (the top number) of the fraction remains the same but the denominator (the bottom number) changes, and thus the overall concentration value goes down.

For example, a simple fraction like 10/5 becomes 10/10 when diluted (notice the top number stays the same but the bottom number doubles):

$$\frac{10 \text{ mg}}{5 \text{ mL}} = 2 \text{ mg/mL}$$

$$\frac{10 \text{ mg}}{10 \text{ mL}} = 1 \text{ mg/mL}$$

In this example, the concentration was cut in half by doubling the volume in which the drug is dissolved.

Pharmacy technicians can help pharmacists in figuring out either how much diluent needs to be added to either to get the volume needed or how much to add to get to the concentration desired.

EXAMPLE

Solving the Volume Needed to Achieve Desired Concentration

You receive a prescription that calls for one pound (1 lb) of 15% urea in ammonium lactate lotion. Your pharmacist tells you that it is difficult to use urea crystals (powder) to make this and that she would like to use a commercially-available product and dilute it down. You go to the shelf and find that the only urea cream in the pharmacy is 40% in 85 g tubes. How much of the 40% cream do you need to add to the ammonium lactate lotion to get one pound of 15% urea lotion?

Note: One pound (1 lb) is approximately 454 g.

Step 1: Determine how much urea is in 454 g of 15% urea in ammonium lactate by setting up an equation.

$$\frac{15 \text{ g urea}}{100 \text{ g mixture}} = \frac{Y \text{ g urea}}{454 \text{ g mixture}}$$

Step 2: Cross multiply to solve for the unknown (Y).

$$100 \text{ g mixture} \times Y \text{ g urea} = 15 \text{ g urea} \times 454 \text{ g mixture}$$

$$\frac{100 \, \cancel{\text{g mixture}} \times Y \text{ g urea}}{100 \, \cancel{\text{g mixture}}} = \frac{15 \text{ g urea} \times 454 \, \cancel{\text{g mixture}}}{100 \, \cancel{\text{g mixture}}}$$

$$Y \text{ g urea} = \frac{15 \times 454 \text{ g urea}}{100}$$

$$Y \text{ g urea} = \frac{6,810 \text{ g urea}}{100}$$

$$Y \text{ g urea} = 68.1 \text{ g urea}$$

Step 3: Determine how much 40% urea is needed to provide 68.1 g of urea by setting up an equation. Commercial product = cp

$$\frac{40 \text{ g urea}}{100 \text{ g cp}} = \frac{68.1 \text{ g urea}}{Z \text{ g cp}}$$

Step 4: Cross multiply to solve for the unknown (Z).

40 g urea x Z g cp = 100 g cp x 68.1 g urea

$$\frac{40 \text{ g urea} \times Z \text{ g cp}}{40 \text{ g urea}} = \frac{100 \text{ g cp} \times 68.1 \text{ g urea}}{40 \text{ g urea}}$$

$$Z \text{ g cp} = \frac{100 \times 68.1 \text{ g cp}}{40}$$

$$Z \text{ g cp} = \frac{6,810 \text{ g cp}}{40}$$

$$Z \text{ g cp} = 170.25 \text{ g cp}$$

Step 5: Determine how much ammonium lactate lotion is needed if 170.25 g of commercial product is added.

454 g mixture – 170.25 g commercial product = 283.75 g ammonium lactate lotion

You present a recipe to your pharmacist calling for adding 170.25 g of 40% urea cream (commercial product) to 283.75 g of ammonium lactate lotion to make 454 g of 15% urea in ammonium lactate. She checks your math, agrees, and asks you to start weighing out the commercial urea cream while she finds a one pound dispensing jar.

Mixing Mixtures of Different Concentrations

When the concentration required to fill a prescription is not commercially available, but is somewhere between two commercially-available concentrations, a pharmacy technician can help a pharmacist mix the two commercially-available products together to get to the desired concentration. There are two ways to represent this mathematically that both lead to the same result; one method is called the algebraic method and the other method is called the alligation method. Pharmacy technicians may use whichever of these methods makes the most sense to them but must be familiar with both methods. Both require a little memorization (or a convenient reminder card) to set up the calculation correctly. The algebraic method requires knowing at least two formulas, and the alligation method requires knowing how to set up the grid used in this method. This section contains the many details to getting this process right.

To use either method, the units of the concentrations must all be the same (e.g., mg/mL). If the units are not the same (e.g., mg/mL and g/dL), convert one of the concentrations to match the units of the other before beginning.

> Tip: the concentration of the finished mixture cannot be higher than the highest-concentration ingredient and cannot be lower than the lowest-concentration ingredient; the finished concentration MUST be between the concentrations of the two commercial ingredient mixtures.

Mixing Mixtures: The Algebraic Method

If the concentration and volume of the finished mixture are known, and the concentrations of the commercial ingredients are known, the following formulas can be used to find how much of each commercial ingredient is necessary to reach the finished concentration at the finished volume.

The volume or weight of the higher-concentration ingredient needed is:

$$\frac{F - L}{H - L} \times V$$

The volume or weight of the lower-concentration ingredient needed is:

$$\frac{H - F}{H - L} \times V$$

F = Concentration of the FINISHED mixture
L = Concentration of the LOWER-concentration commercial ingredient
H = Concentration of the HIGHER-concentration commercial ingredient
V = Volume (or weight) of the FINISHED mixture

Mixing Mixtures: The Alligation Method

A visual representation of the equations used in the algebraic method, called the alligation method, looks like a "Tic-Tac-Toe" board and is setup as follows:

F = Concentration of the FINISHED mixture
L = Concentration of the LOWER-concentration commercial ingredient
H = Concentration of the HIGHER-concentration commercial ingredient
V = Volume (or weight) of the FINISHED mixture

Step 1 H		Step 2 F − L = PARTS H	Step 5 PARTS H ÷ Total PARTS = %H	Step 7 %H x V
	Step 1 F	Step 1 V	Step 4 PARTS H + PARTS L = Total PARTS	Step 9 %H x V + %L x V
Step 1 L		Step 3 H − F = PARTS L	Step 6 PARTS L ÷ Total PARTS = %L	Step 8 %L x V

To complete this method draw the grid and, follow these steps:
1. Enter the known values of H, L, F and V.
2. Determine F minus L and enter as PARTS H.
3. Determine H minus F and enter as PARTS L.
4. Add PARTS H (as found in step 2) and PARTS L (as found in step 3) and enter it as Total PARTS.
5. Determine PARTS H (as found in step 2) divided by Total PARTS (as found in step 4) and enter it as %H.
6. Determine PARTS L (as found in step 3) divided by Total PARTS (as found in step 4) and enter it as %L.
7. Multiply %H (as found in step 5) and V to determine the volume or weight needed of the lower concentration commercial ingredient. This is the amount of the lower concentrated product you would add to the mixture.
8. Multiply %L (as found in step 6) and V to determine the volume or weight needed of the higher concentration commercial ingredient. This is the amount of the higher concentrated product you would add to the mixture.
9. Add the answers to step 7 (%H x V) and 8 (%L x V) as a double check to ensure you performed the operation successfully. The sum MUST equal V, or the volume of the finished mixture.

EXAMPLE
Determining a Recipe Via the Algebraic and Alligation Methods

You receive a prescription for 454 g of triamcinolone acetonide 0.05% cream to treat an itching rash that is all over the patient's body. Triamcinolone acetonide isn't commercially available as a 0.05% cream; it comes as a 0.1% cream and 0.025% cream. Your pharmacist looks to you to enter the compound into the computer system and so you must figure out a recipe for this prescription.

Using the Algebraic Method:

Step 1: Determine the weight of the higher concentration commercial ingredient (0.1% cream) that is needed.

$$\frac{F - L}{H - I} \times V, \text{ where } F = 0.05\%, L = 0.025\%, H = 0.1\%,$$
$$V = 454 \text{ g}$$

$$\frac{0.05\% - 0.025\%}{0.1\% - 0.025\%} \times 454 \text{ g}$$

Convert each percent to a decimal number.

$$\frac{0.0005 - 0.00025}{0.001 - 0.00025} \times 454 \text{ g}$$

$$\frac{0.00025}{0.00075} \times 454 \text{ g} = 151.3 \text{ g}$$

Therefore, 151.3 g of the higher concentrated commercial ingredient (0.1% cream) is needed.

Step 2: Determine the weight of the lower concentration commercial product (0.025% cream) that is needed.

$$\frac{H - F}{H - L} \times V$$

$$\frac{0.1\% - 0.05\%}{0.1\% - 0.025\%} \times 454 \text{ g}$$

$$\frac{0.0005}{0.00075} \times 454 \text{ g} = 302.66 \text{ g} \text{ rounded to } 302.7 \text{ g}$$

Therefore, 302.7 g of the lower concentration commercial product (0.025% cream) is needed.

Step 3: Add the weights for each ingredient to be sure the ingredients add up to the finished weight.

151.3 g (higher concentration cream) + 302.7 g (lower concentration cream) = 454 g (total volume of finished product)

Using the Alligation Method

H = 0.1		0.05 – 0.025 = 0.025 (PARTS H)	0.025 ÷ 0.075 = 0.3333 (%H)	0.3333 x 454 = 151.3182 g rounded to 151.3 g
	F = 0.05	V = 454 g	0.025 + 0.05 = 0.075 (Total PARTS)	151.3 g + 302.7 g = 454 g = (V)
L = 0.025		0.1 – 0.05 = 0.05 (PARTS L)	0.05 ÷ 0.075 = 0.6667 (%L)	0.6667 x 454 = 302.6818 g rounded to 302.7 g

Using either method, the result is the same.

By adding 151.3 g of 0.1% triamcinolone acetonide cream to 302.7 g of 0.025% triamcinolone cream, 454 g of 0.05% triamcinolone acetonide cream can be compounded. Your pharmacist verifies your calculation, agrees, and asks you to start weighing out the 0.025% cream.

Manipulating Concentration-Based Medication Orders

Common antibiotics, such as amoxicillin and azithromycin, come as powders for suspension such that, when the specified amount of water is added, the suspension is at a standard concentration. Knowing these standard concentrations, prescribers will adjust the volume given at each dose to provide the total amount of drug desired. Sometimes, however, one of the concentrations is unavailable (because of a manufacturer's backorder or a pharmacy simply being out) and a pharmacy technician must work with his or her pharmacist to manipulate the amount given at each dose based on the available concentrations. Note that the weight of drug given at each dose does not change (e.g., 400 mg); only the volume given at each dose changes (e.g., 5 mL becomes 3.5 mL).

EXAMPLE
Adjusting for Difference in Concentration

A prescription is written as follows:

Amoxicillin 400 mg/5 mL. Give patient 3.5 mL three times daily for ten days. Dispense a sufficient quantity. No refills.

You go to the shelf and find that you are all out of 400 mg/5 mL amoxicillin. So, you look for the next closest strength and find that you do have plenty of 250 mg/5 mL amoxicillin. After adjusting for this difference in concentration, what amount will be distributed to the patient?

Step 1: Determine how much amoxicillin (in milligrams) goes into each dose in the original prescription.

$$\frac{3.5 \text{ mL}}{\text{dose}} \times \frac{400 \text{ mg}}{5 \text{ mL}} = \frac{280 \text{ mg}}{\text{dose}}$$

Step 2: Determine what volume of 250 mg/5 mL amoxicillin will provide a 280 mg dose.

$$\frac{250 \text{ mg}}{5 \text{ mL}} = \frac{280 \text{ mg}}{Z}$$

$$250 \text{ mg} \times Z = 5 \text{ mL} \times 280 \text{ mg}$$

$$\frac{\cancel{250 \text{ mg}} \times Z}{\cancel{250 \text{ mg}}} = \frac{5 \text{ mL} \times 280 \cancel{\text{ mg}}}{250 \cancel{\text{ mg}}}$$

$$Z = \frac{5 \text{ mL} \times 280}{250}$$

$$Z = \frac{1,400 \text{ mL}}{250}$$

$$Z = 5.6 \text{ mL}$$

Step 3: Determine the total amount of 250 mg/ 5 mL amoxicillin required to provide all of the doses.

$$\frac{5.6 \text{ mL}}{\text{dose}} \times \frac{3 \text{ doses}}{\text{day}} \times 10 \text{ days} =$$

$$\frac{5.6 \text{ mL}}{\cancel{\text{dose}}} \times \frac{3 \cancel{\text{doses}}}{\cancel{\text{day}}} \times 10 \cancel{\text{days}} = 168 \text{ mL}$$

On a separate piece of paper, you write out the "new prescription" that will be attached to the prescriber's original order and provide it to your pharmacist to verify and approve. This "new prescription" reads:

Amoxicillin 250 mg/5 mL. Give the patient 5.6 mL by mouth three times daily for ten days. Dispense: a minimum of 168 mL. No refills.

References

1. "Diluent." *Mosby's Dictionary of Complementary and Alternative Medicine*. Philadelphia: Elsevier Health Sciences, 2005. *Credo Reference*. Web. 15 December 2009.

2. "Heterogeneous." *Academic Press Dictionary of Science and Technology*. Oxford: Elsevier Science & Technology, 1992. *Credo Reference*. Web. 15 December 2009.

3. "Homogeneous." *McGraw-Hill Dictionary of Scientific and Technical Terms*. New York: McGraw-Hill, 2003. *Credo Reference*. Web. 15 December 2009.

4. "Mixture." *The American Heritage Science Dictionary*. Boston: Houghton Mifflin, 2005. *Credo Reference*. Web. 15 December 2009.

5. "Solute." *The American Heritage Science Dictionary*. Boston: Houghton Mifflin, 2005. *Credo Reference*. Web. 15 December 2009.

6. "Solution." *The American Heritage Science Dictionary*. Boston: Houghton Mifflin, 2005. *Credo Reference*. Web. 15 December 2009.

7. "Solvent." *The American Heritage Science Dictionary*. Boston: Houghton Mifflin, 2005. *Credo Reference*. Web. 15 December 2009.

8. "Suspension." *The American Heritage Science Dictionary*. Boston: Houghton Mifflin, 2005. *Credo Reference*. Web. 15 December 2009.

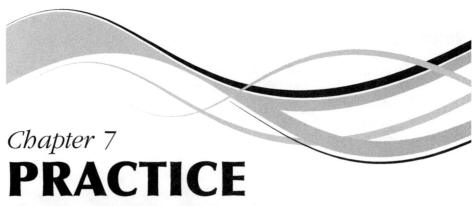

Chapter 7
PRACTICE PROBLEMS

1.   How much desoximetasone is in 100 g of 0.25% desoximetasone ointment (in grams)?

2.   How much ketoconazole (in grams) is in 8 oz of 15% compounded ketoconazole lotion?

3.   A prescription is written: Give Stacy promethazine with codeine 6.25 mg/10 mg/5 mL. How much codeine is in 120 mL of promethazine with codeine 6.25 mg/10 mg/5 mL?

4.   How much ethanol is in 480 mL of a solution of 82% ethanol (in milliliters)?

5.   An IV bag currently contains 150 mL of 40% KCl; the recipe provided to you says to add 50 mL of sterile water to the bag. What is the final concentration of KCl in the bag?

6.   The pharmacy stocks a 20% solution of oxybutinin and you receive a prescription for 120 mL of 4% oxybutinin; write a recipe for this prescription that involves diluting down the stock solution with water to the required concentration.

7.   How many grams of NaCl are in 500 mL of normal (0.9%) saline (saline is NaCl dissolved in water)?

8.   Write an appropriate recipe (provide the weight or volume of each ingredient) for compounding 480 mL of a 0.125 mg/mL hydrocortisone | 5.2 mg/5 mL tetracycline | 6.25% nystatin liquid | 93.5% diphenhydramine mixture used to treat mouth sores. Calculate how much diphenhydramine is needed; however, note that, in practice, diphenhydramine is considered the base of this compound so enough diphenhydramine will be added to bring the total volume up to 480 mL after all other ingredients are added.

9.   What is the final weight of a 2% salicylic acid ointment made by adding petroleum jelly to 15 g of 10% salicylic acid ointment?

10. In a country of 1.2 billion people, there are 17 people with typhoid fever. How could one express the concentration of typhoid fever in the country in parts per million (ppm)?

11. You receive a prescription that calls for adding sterile water to 150 mL of 15% acetic acid until 500 mL of solution is achieved. What is the final concentration of acetic acid after the dilution is performed?

12. If an air filter allows only 0.1 ppb dust particles (and 100% of air) through it into a sterile area, and there are 5.7 billion particles (dust and air) hitting the air filter every second, how long will it take before the filter allows 100 dust particles through?

13. A 40% solution of isopropyl alcohol has been diluted to 100 mL of 20% isopropyl alcohol by adding sterile water. How much of the starting 40% solution must have been present to compound this final concentration?

14. A massage therapist calls the pharmacy and asks if the pharmacist can mix up a batch of peppermint massage oil for him. Your pharmacist agrees and asks you, her technician, to collect the ingredients and mix up the batch. You find that you have a concentrated 80% oil of peppermint stock bottle with 480 mL of oil in it. The massage therapist needs a 25% oil packaged in 240 mL bottles; how many 240 mL bottles can you make with your stock bottle by diluting with jojoba oil?

15. A pharmacist asks a pharmacy technician to verify that his calculations are correct for the compound that he is about to mix up. You examine his recipe and label and find that an error has been made. Based on the following information, where is the error? What is (are) the corrected value(s)?

    The prescription reads:
    For Heather, mix:
    > 120 g of 2% ketoconazole cream
    > 90 g of 1% hydrocortisone cream
    > Quantity sufficient coal tar to make the final compound 2% coal tar solution
    > Quantity sufficient of a cream base to provide 454 g of finished compound

    > Apply to red patches three times daily as needed for psoriasis. 454 g. 5 Refills.

    Your pharmacist's recipe reads:
    Mix:
    > 120 g of 2% ketoconazole cream
    > 90 g of 1% hydrocortisone cream
    > 9.08 g of coal tar solution
    > 234.92 g of cream base

    Your pharmacist's label for the jar reads:
    > ketoconazole/hydrocortisone/coal tar 2%/1%/2% in a cream base.

    Have Heather apply to red patches three times daily as needed for psoriasis. 454 g. 5 Refills.

16. You receive an order to dissolve menthol crystals into sterile water to make 480 mL of 8% menthol solution. Shortly after compounding this prescription, the nurse calls back and apologizes for making an error; the prescription was for 3% menthol. How much sterile water must be added to your compound to produce at least 480 mL of 3% menthol?

17. A recipe for a compound asks the preparer to add 20 g ketoconazole into 473 mL ammonium lactate lotion. What percent of the resulting compound is ketoconazole?

18. A prescription for Chad calls for triamcinolone injectable suspension 10 mg/mL to be diluted down to 0.125 mg/mL by adding distilled water (this is used to treat mouth sores). How much triamcinolone suspension and how much water must be added to make 480 mL of the final product?

19. A prescription arrives at the pharmacy and calls for 0.089% betamethasone diproprionate lotion to be applied to patient Dana's arms three times daily for 30 days. The specified quantity is two pounds (908 g). Betamethasone diproprionate lotion only comes as a 0.1% and 0.05% commercial product. Write a recipe for this compound.

20. A prescription calls for 100 mL of 30% ethanol to be compounded from 25% ethanol and 50% ethanol. Write a recipe for this compound.

21. A prescription to treat "strep throat" is written: Give Kristi 3.5 mL of a 250 mg/5 mL cefdinir suspension twice daily for 10 days. Upon reaching the shelf, you find that you are out of 250 mg/5 mL suspension but you have plenty of the 125 mg/5 mL suspension. Write out how this prescription would look using the 125 mg/5 mL suspension.

22. Your pharmacist presents you with a recipe for a compound that calls for grinding ibuprofen tablets (standard strengths are 200 mg, 400 mg and 800 mg tablets) and adding the resulting powder to petroleum jelly to form a topical ibuprofen ointment. If the 800 mg tablets are cheaper (by the milligram) than the 400 mg tablets, and the 400 mg tablets are cheaper than the 200 mg tablets, how many of which strength tablets must be ground to make 454 g of 30% ibuprofen ointment to make the lowest cost compound possible?

23. What is the weight (in milligrams) of active ingredient present in 30 g of a 7% ointment?

24. According to the Carbon Dioxide Information Analysis Center, there are 384.8 ppm of carbon dioxide currently in our atmosphere as of April 20, 2010 (cdi-ac.ornl.gov). If 999,000 parts of the atmosphere is nitrogen gases and oxygen gas, how much of the atmosphere is made up of chemicals other than the three main gases (carbon dioxide, nitrogen and oxygen)?

25. You receive a prescription to compound 5% coal tar and 2% salicylic acid added to commercially available 0.005% calcipotriene cream (120 g tube) to treat psoriasis. If coal tar comes as a 200 mg/mL solution, how much coal tar solution (in milliliters) must be added to the 120 g tube of calcipotriene to make final compound be 5% coal tar?

26. You receive a prescription that calls for giving 500 mg four times daily for seven days to a 12 year old with a mild penicillin allergy and a minor sinus infection. The patient's father is concerned that his son will not do well swallowing capsules and asks if there's a liquid available. You find that you have a 100 mL and a 200 mL bottle of 250 mg/5 mL cephalexin powder for suspension on the shelf. What is the total volume (in mL) that you will need to provide the full course of therapy, and do you have enough bottles in the pharmacy to provide the full course of therapy or will you need to send the patient home with what you have and order more?

27. You receive a prescription for Sally Scratchins for an itch relieving topical cream with this recipe: combine 8 g 1% hydrocortisone, 14 g 1% diphenhydramine and acid mantle up to 30 g. How much diphenhydramine is in the final compound (expressed in grams)?

28. One of your fellow technicians sets out to make a compound when she begins to question herself. Before presenting her recipe to your pharmacist, she asks you to check her work because it just doesn't seem right. Based on the prescription presented, does the recipe she devised make sense?

> Patient: Art Wright
> DOB: 05/17/2007
>
> > Compound: Naproxen 25 mg/mL & Folic Acid 0.1 mg/mL
> > Give Art one teaspoonful twice daily
> > Q.S. 30 days / Ref: PRN
> >
> > > Dr. N. Ced

Your colleague's recipe: Grind 300 folic acid 1 mg tablets and mix with 450 mL of naproxen 125 mg/5 mL suspension through a mortar.

29. The local headache clinic calls and asks if you can make a nasal spray of mupirocin and saline for a patient. You inform them that you don't see a recipe in your book of compounds but that your pharmacist says that she will help you write a new recipe and that the pharmacy can, indeed, complete this request. When the prescription arrives, it calls for adding 4.6 g of mupirocin ointment into 88 mL of 0.9% nasal saline with the compound to be dispensed in a clean nasal spray bottle. The mupirocin dissolves completely so the final compound's volume will be 88 mL. Your pharmacist starts writing up the recipe and asks you to prepare the label for the final compound. What is the concentration you will list for the mupirocin on the label (in mg/mL)?

30. A prescription calls for 0.68% capsaicin cream to be applied to the skin after shingles sores have subsided but where pain persists. The physician believes that 60 g is appropriate for this patient to last one month and asks you to dispense a one-month supply. Unfortunately, your pharmacy only stocks 0.75% and 0.035% capsaicin. Your pharmacist reminds you that you were trained in the alligation method for combining mixtures and asks you to write him a recipe for mixing up this compound. What is the recipe to fill the prescription with the ingredients available (using the alligation method)?

Chapter 8

INTRAVENOUS FLOW RATE AND COMPOUNDING INTRAVENOUS PRODUCTS

By Karen Woods Miron, R.Ph.

Learning Objectives

Upon completion of this chapter, the technician should be able to:
- understand the difference between a hydration solution and a solution used to deliver medication.
- determine the flow rate of intravenous solutions based on time.
- determine flow rate based on concentration of solution.
- understand the impact of significant powder volume when reconstituting medications.
- understand the importance of calculating final concentration of IV solutions.
- perform calculations involving reconstitution of dry powders.

Introduction

Parenteral and **intravenous** (IV) are terms used to describe a method of medication administration that delivers medication directly into a patient's vein. IV administration can be used as a means of hydrating a patient (adding volume to their blood stream), a means of administering medications to a patient or as a means of giving a patient nutrition.

For **hydration** purposes, physicians generally order a volume of fluid per hour.

These are relatively simple calculations, multiplying the amount of fluid ordered per hour by 24 hours in a day so that you can calculate the total number of IV bags that a patient needs in a 24-hour period of time. Hydration IVs are usually dispensed as 1 Liter (1,000 mL) bags.

When **medication** is to be administered via the IV route, the order may be written in a variety of ways:

- As a total amount of medication to be given
- As an amount of medication to be given over a certain amount of time
- As an amount of medication per kg of body weight per an amount of time

When medications are administered via the intravenous route, it is important to understand the concentration of medication that is being administered.

For nutritional therapy, intravenous solutions containing protein, dextrose, electrolytes and sometimes fat are compounded in the pharmacy. These solutions are referred to as **Total Parenteral Nutrition** or TPN.

Intravenous Flow Rate

The flow rate of an intravenous solution is the volume of solution given to a patient over a period of time. This is generally expressed as mL/hr.

Basic intravenous solutions of sodium chloride, dextrose or combinations of these ingredients are used to hydrate patients. Depending on the patient's physical needs, age or size, the physician will usually order these solutions in milliliters per hour (mL/hr). It is important to know how long each 1,000 mL bag will last; this will help you determine when the next bag will be needed and how many bags of solution will be needed in a 24-hour period.

EXAMPLE
Calculating Daily Volume of Fluid

If a large volume IV is ordered to flow at 125 mL/hr, determine the amount of fluid that will be administered in one day.

The following formula is used:
daily volume of fluid (mL/day) = flow rate (mL/hr) x 24 hr/day

Step 1: Insert the known values into the formula.

$$\text{daily volume of fluid (mL/day)} = \frac{125 \text{ mL}}{\text{hr}} \times \frac{24 \text{ hr}}{\text{day}}$$

daily volume of fluid (mL/day) =

$$\frac{125 \text{ mL}}{\text{hr}} \times \frac{24 \text{ hr}}{\text{day}} = \frac{125 \text{ mL} \times 24}{\text{day}}$$

INTRAVENOUS FLOW RATE AND COMPOUNDING INTRAVENOUS PRODUCTS *Chapter 8*

$$\text{daily volume of fluid (mL/day)} = \frac{3{,}000 \text{ mL}}{\text{day}}$$

Therefore, 3,000 mL of fluid will be administered in one day at 125 mL/hr.

EXAMPLE
Calculating the Number of 1,000 mL Bags of Fluid Needed in 24 Hours

Using this formula and information from the previous example, determine the number of 1,000 mL bags in 24 hours.

Number of bags needed per day =
Total volume in mL per day ÷ 1,000 mL/bag

Step 1: Insert known values into the formula and solve.

$$\text{\# of bags needed/day} = \frac{3{,}000 \text{ mL}}{\text{day}} \div \frac{1{,}000 \text{ mL}}{\text{bag}}$$

# of bags needed/day =

$$\frac{3{,}000 \text{ mL}}{\text{day}} \times \frac{\text{bag}}{1{,}000 \text{ mL}} = \frac{3{,}000 \text{ bags}}{1{,}000 \text{ day}} = 3 \text{ bags/day}$$

Most technicians will memorize the following common flow rates for hydration IVs:

Rate	Total Volume in 24 hours:	# of 1,000 mL bags/24 hours
150 mL/hour	3,600 mL	3.6 bags
125 mL/hour	3,000 mL	3 bags
100 mL/hour	2,400 mL	2.4 bags
80 mL/hr	1,920 mL	2 bags
50 mL/hr	1,200 mL	1.2 bags
42 mL/hr	1,008 mL	1 bag

Intravenous Flow Rate by Administration Set

Intravenous flow rates must be accurately determined to ensure that patients receive an appropriate dose of medication over a specified time frame. Factors to consider when calculating IV flow rates include the total volume of the IV solution, the length of administration time and the method of administering the infusion.

Most institutions use special IV pumps to administer medications via the intravenous route. Most pumps will have their matching tubing sets to guarantee an accurate flow rate. A few institutions still use tubing that has a drip chamber where you must calculate the capacity of the tubing to determine the flow rate. Smaller volumes of fluid are usually referred to as IV piggybacks (IVPB) because they are "piggybacked" or infused through the fluid of a large volume IV using the same administration set. Using flow rates, one can calculate the volume of fluid and/or the amount of drug a patient will receive over a certain period of time. In IV flow rate calculations, hours are typically represented by the abbreviations "h" or "hr," minutes are represented by "min" and drops are represented by "gtt."

The most common IV administration sets are calibrated to deliver 10 or 60 gtt/mL, but one should always verify the type of administration set that will be used before performing calculations to determine the rate of delivery. The basic mathematical principles involved in IV flow rate calculations frequently involve the concepts used in ratios and proportions. The following formulas are used to perform flow rate calculations.

daily volume of fluid (mL/day) = flow rate (mL/hr) x 24 hr/day

$$\text{IV flow rate} = \frac{\text{dose desired}}{\text{concentration of IV}}$$

If using tubing with a drip chamber, use this formula to calculate flow rate:

$$\text{IV flow rate (gtt/min)} = \frac{\text{gtt}}{\text{mL}} \times \frac{\text{mL}}{\text{min}}$$

EXAMPLE
Calculating IV Flow Rates in Drops/Minute

Determine the flow rate for 50 mL of an antibiotic IVPB infused over 60 minutes if the administration set is calibrated to deliver 20 gtt/mL.

Step 1: Insert the known values into the formula and solve.

$$\text{IV flow rate (gtt/min)} = \frac{\text{gtt}}{\text{mL}} \times \frac{\text{mL}}{\text{min}}$$

$$\text{IV flow rate (gtt/min)} = \frac{20 \text{ gtt}}{\text{mL}} \times \frac{50 \text{ mL}}{60 \text{ min}}$$

$$\text{IV flow rate (gtt/min)} = \frac{20 \text{ gtt}}{\text{mL}} \times \frac{50 \text{ mL}}{60 \text{ min}}$$

$$\text{IV flow rate (gtt/min)} = \frac{1{,}000 \text{ gtt}}{60 \text{ min}}$$

$$\text{IV flow rate (gtt/min)} = 17 \text{ gtt/min}$$

Therefore, a 50 mL IVPB infused over 60 minutes, utilizing an administration set to deliver 20 gtt/mL, will have an IV flow rate of 17 gtt/min.

Calculating IV Flow Rates for Solutions Containing Medications

EXAMPLE
Calculating Flow Rate When an Exact Amount of Medication is to be Given

An order is received for 2 grams of vancomycin in 500 mL of 0.9% NaCl to be given over 2 hours. What is the flow rate of the solution?

Note: Flow rate is volume over time; in this example the amount of medication isn't necessary to determine flow rate.

$$\text{Flow rate} = \frac{\text{Volume}}{\text{Time}}$$

$$\text{Flow rate} = \frac{500 \text{ mL}}{2 \text{ hr}} = \frac{250 \text{ mL}}{1 \text{ hr}}$$

EXAMPLE
Calculating Flow Rate Based on Drug Concentration

Your hospital stocks a standard heparin solution of 25,000 units in 500 mL of 5% dextrose. The physician orders 800 units heparin/hour. Determine the correct rate of infusion in mL/h.

Step 1: Determine the concentration of the solution by dividing the total amount of drug by the total volume.

$$\text{concentration of IV} = \frac{\text{total amount of drug}}{\text{total volume}} =$$

$$\frac{25,000 \text{ units}}{500 \text{ mL}} = 50 \text{ units/mL}$$

Step 2: Insert the known values into the formula to determine flow rate.

$$\text{IV flow rate} = \frac{\text{dose desired}}{\text{concentration of IV}}$$

$$\text{IV flow rate} = \frac{800 \text{ units/hr}}{50 \text{ units/mL}} = \frac{800 \text{ units}}{\text{hr}} \div \frac{50 \text{ units}}{\text{mL}}$$

$$\text{IV flow rate} = \frac{800 \text{ \sout{units}}}{\text{hr}} \times \frac{\text{mL}}{50 \text{ \sout{units}}}$$

$$\text{IV flow rate} = \frac{800 \text{ mL}}{50 \text{ hr}} = 16 \text{ mL/hr}$$

Therefore, heparin 25,000 units in 500 mL 5% dextrose should be infused at 16 mL/hr to deliver 800 units/hr.

Calculating Flow Rate Based on Dose Over Time

Hospitalized patients, particularly those in intensive or critical care units, are often given medication through a continuous IV infusion that is dosed on an exact amount of medication in a specified period of time.

The following formula is helpful when performing these types of calculations.

IV flow rate (mL/hr) = $\dfrac{\text{dose}}{\text{hr}} \times \dfrac{\text{volume of IV}}{\text{concentration of IV}}$

EXAMPLE
Calculating IV Flow Rate in mL/hr
When a Set Dose is Involved

The pharmacy supplies morphine in a standard IV solution of 5 mg/mL. The doctor orders morphine continuous infusion of 8 mg/hour. What would the IV flow rate be in mL/hr?

Step 1: Insert the known values into the formula and solve.

IV flow rate (mL/hr) = $\dfrac{8 \text{ mg}}{\text{hr}} \times \dfrac{1 \text{ mL}}{5 \text{ mg}}$

IV flow rate (mL/hr) = $\dfrac{8 \text{ \cancel{mg}}}{\text{hr}} \times \dfrac{1 \text{ mL}}{5 \text{ \cancel{mg}}}$

IV flow rate (mL/hr) = $\dfrac{8 \text{ mL}}{5 \text{ hr}}$

IV flow rate (mL/hr) = 1.6 mL/hr

Therefore, the IV flow rate to deliver 8 mg per hour would be 1.6 mL/hr.

Physicians may order the dose of IV medications based upon the patient's weight. When this occurs, the following formula, which is a slight modification of the afore-mentioned formula, should be utilized to determine the IV flow rate. In this example, the dose was ordered per minute, so that also has to be factored into the equation.

IV flow rate (mL/hr) =

$\dfrac{\text{dose}}{\text{kg/min}} \times \text{weight in kg} \times \dfrac{\text{volume of IV}}{\text{concentration of IV}} \times \dfrac{60 \text{ min}}{1 \text{ hr}}$

EXAMPLE

Calculating IV Flow Rate in mL/hr When a Dosage Based Upon Weight is Involved

The doctor orders a milrinone dose of 0.375 mcg/kg/min. You stock a pre-mixed solution containing 200 mcg/mL in 200 mL bags. (40,000 mcg/200 mL) What would the IV flow rate be in mL/hr for a patient weighing 70 kg?

Step 1: Insert the known values into the formula and solve. (It should be noted that the concentration and dose/kg must be in the same metric units; in this case both are in mcg.)

IV flow rate (mL/hr) =

$$\frac{0.375 \text{ mcg}}{\text{kg/min}} \times 70 \text{ kg} \times \frac{200 \text{ mL}}{40,000 \text{ mcg}} \times \frac{60 \text{ min}}{1 \text{ hr}}$$

IV flow rate (mL/hr) =

$$\frac{0.375 \text{ \sout{mcg}}}{\text{\sout{kg/min}}} \times 70 \text{ \sout{kg}} \times \frac{200 \text{ mL}}{40,000 \text{ \sout{mcg}}} \times \frac{60 \text{ \sout{min}}}{1 \text{ hr}}$$

$$\text{IV flow rate (mL/hr)} = \frac{0.375 \times 70 \times 200 \times 60 \text{ mL}}{40,000 \times 1 \text{ hr}}$$

$$\text{IV flow rate (mL/hr)} = \frac{315,000 \text{ mL}}{40,000 \text{ hr}}$$

IV flow rate (mL/hr) = 7.875 mL/hr

Therefore, the IV flow rate to deliver 0.375 mcg per kg per minute would be 7.875 mL/hr, rounded to 7.9 mL/hr for most delivery systems.

Reconstitution of Dry Powders

Some drugs, IV parenterals, oral suspensions, etc., are not stable for long time periods in their solution form, so they are packaged by manufacturers as dry powders to increase their shelf life. These types of medications must be dissolved in solution prior to dispensing. The solution used to dissolve the dry powder is referred to as the **diluent**. The amount of space occupied by the dry powder is known as **powder volume**. Powder volume can also be defined as the difference between the amount of diluent and the final volume of the medication in solution.

If the powder volume is negligible, the volume of diluent used will be the same as the intended final volume of the reconstituted solution. However, if the dry powder has significant bulk and contributes to the final volume of the reconstituted solution, then it must be subtracted from the diluent volume to ensure the correct concentration of the resulting reconstituted solution. The following formulas explain this relationship.

diluent volume = final volume – powder volume

powder volume = final volume – diluent volume

EXAMPLE
Determining Diluent Volume

If an antibiotic in its dry powder form occupies 1.2 mL and the total volume of its reconstituted solution is 10 mL, determine the amount of diluent needed to prepare the solution.

Step 1: Insert the known values into the formula and solve.

diluent volume = 10 mL – 1.2 mL

diluent volume = 8.8 mL

Therefore, 8.8 mL of diluent added to the 1.2 mL of antibiotic powder will result in 10 mL of reconstituted solution.

EXAMPLE
Determining Diluent Volume

If you were asked to dilute that vial of powder to 100 mL, how much diluent would you add?

Step 1: Insert the known values into the formula and solve.

Diluent volume = 100 mL – 1.2 mL

Diluent volume = 98.8 mL

Therefore, 98.8 mL of diluent added to the 1.2 mL of antibiotic powder will result in 100 mL of reconstituted solution.

EXAMPLE
Determining Powder Volume

If the final volume of a reconstituted suspension should be 150 mL and the instructions indicate to add 117 mL of water to the dry powder, determine the powder volume of the medication.

Step 1: Insert the known values into the formula and solve.

powder volume = 150 mL – 117 mL

powder volume = 33 mL

Therefore, the powder volume is 33 mL.

Chapter 8
PRACTICE PROBLEMS

1. If an IV fluid is ordered at 125 mL/hr, how much fluid will the patient receive in a 24-hour period?

2. The physician orders dextrose 5% in water at 62 cc/hr. How much solution will be administered each day?

3. The doctor orders heparin 25,000 units in 250 mL dextrose 5% in water to infuse at 1,400 units/hr. What is the correct rate of infusion in mL/hr?

4. The doctor changes the dose of heparin to be administered at 900 units per hour using the same IV concentration of heparin 25,000 units in 250 mL. What is the new rate of infusion in mL/hr?

5. What is the flow rate (mL/hr) for 50 mL of an antibiotic IVPB infused over 60 minutes?

6. If a physician orders 70 units of insulin in 50 mL of 0.9% NaCl to be administered over 30 minutes, what is the flow rate in mL/hour?

7. Using the information from problem #6, how much insulin will be delivered in the first 20 minutes of the infusion?

8. Determine the infusion time of 1 L of D5W if a control flow set is at 18 mL/hr.

9. Determine the infusion time of 500 mL of 0.9% NaCl IV if an infusion is ordered to run at 125 mL/hr.

10. The pharmacy stocks a premixed lidocaine IV containing 2 g of lidocaine in 500 mL of D5W. The physician orders a lidocaine drip at an infusion rate of 4 mg/min. What is the IV flow rate in mL/hr?

11. The doctor orders a nitroprusside drip 50 mg in 250 mL D5W to run 5 mcg/kg/min. For a 60 kg patient, what is the IV flow rate in mL/hr?

12. If the contents of a vial of cefazolin in its dry powder form occupies 1.2 mL and the total volume of its reconstituted solution is 20 mL, what amount of sterile water is needed to prepare the solution?

13. If the final volume of 1 gram amoxicillin reconstituted suspension should be 200 mL and the instructions indicate to add 154 mL of water to the dry powder, what is the powder volume of the amoxicillin?

14. a) If the final volume of vancomycin reconstituted solution should be 10 mL and the instructions indicate to add 9.6 mL of water to the dry powder, what is the powder volume of the vancomycin?
    b) If your IV order is for 1 gram of vancomycin in 250 mL of saline, how much saline will be needed to complete the IV solution?

15. The doctor orders a dopamine drip at 25 mcg/kg/min for an 83 kg woman. Using a standard dopamine solution of 400 mg in 250 mL D5W, what would the IV flow rate be in mL/min?

16. The doctor has ordered 1,000 mL of 0.9% NaCl administered over 8 hours. If the administration set has been calibrated to deliver 60 gtt/mL, at what flow rate (gtt/min) should this IV be administered?

17. An IV piggyback of 50 mL is ordered for a newborn infant at 20 gtt/min. If the administration set is calibrated to deliver 10 gtt/mL, how long will it take to deliver the IV piggyback?

18. Determine the infusion time of 1 L of lactated ringers solution if an infusion set delivering 30 gtt/mL is set at 20 gtt/min.

19. Determine the infusion time in hours of a 2 L hydrating solution if an infusion set delivering 30 gtt/mL is set at 60 gtt/min.

20. If an IV fluid is ordered at 85 mL/hr, how many liters of fluid will the patient receive in a 24-hour period?

21. The doctor orders heparin 25,000 units in 250 mL dextrose 5% in water to infuse at 1,100 units/hr. What is the correct rate of infusion in mL/hr?

22. The doctor orders 500 mL of 0.9% NaCl administered over six hours. If the administration set has been calibrated to deliver 60 gtt/mL, at what flow rate in drops per minute should this IV be administered?

23. What is the flow rate for the 50 mL of an antibiotic IVPB infused over 30 minutes if the administered set is calibrated to deliver 10 gtt/mL?

Use the following scenario to solve problems 24 through 26

The pharmacy stocks penicillin G vials with 5 million units in dry powder form. The reconstitution directions on the vial are as follows:

Desired Concentration (units/mL)	Solvent for Vial (mL)
250,000	18.2
500,000	8.2
750,000	4.8
1,000,000	3.2

24. What volume of dry powder is contained in this container of penicillin G?

25. If the vial was diluted with 8.2 mL of sterile water, what would the volume needed for 2 million units of penicillin G be?

26. If the vial was diluted with 4.8 mL, what would the volume needed for 2 million units of penicillin G be?

Use the following scenario to solve problems 27 and 28.

A 112 lb nursing home patient is prescribed a medication at 0.1 mg/kg/min. The technician prepares an IV with a concentration of 1 g of medication in 1,000 mL of 0.9% NS.

27. How long will the 1,000 mL IV bag last for this patient?

28. If the dose for this patient was 1.5 mg/min, what would the IV flow rate be in mL/hr?

Use the following scenario to solve problems 29 and 30.

The doctor orders 2 mg/kg/hr of phenobarbital IV for a 156-lb patient who is seizing. The pharmacist instructs the technician to put 500 mg of phenobarbital in 250 mL of D5W.

29. What would the IV flow rate be in mL/hr for this preparation?

30. How many hours would one IV bag last?

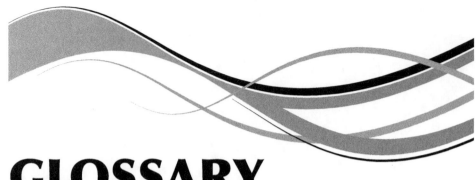

GLOSSARY OF COMMON TERMS RELATED TO PHARMACY CALCULATIONS

Apothecary system

System of weight and liquid measures; the basic apothecary solid (weight) measure is the grain (gr), while the basic fluid (volume) measure is the minim (℥ or ℳ)

Arabic numerals

Numbering system 0, 1, 2, 3, etc.

Avoirdupois system

Ordinary system of weights used in the United States, in which 16 ounces avoirdupois equals a pound; used only for measuring weight; basic unit is the grain (gr)

Body Surface Area (BSA) Nomogram

A "chart" that determines BSA from the weight (mass) and height of the child or adult

Celsius

Temperature measurement that is a component of the metric system; used by most other countries than the United States; freezing point of water is 0 °C and the boiling point is 100 °C

Complex fraction

Fraction in which the numerator and/or denominator are fractions

Conversion

Translating one quantity to another, either in the same or different measurement system

DEA number

Unique number issued by the Drug Enforcement Administration to prescribers who wish to write orders for controlled substances must also be registered with the DEA, as well as facilities and individuals involved with the dispensing of controlled substances

Denominator

Bottom number of the fraction, the whole

Diluent

Inert substance added to source material to thin it to the potency [or concentration] desired

Dosing regimen

Schedule of medication administration; usually includes the name of the drug, the quantity or concentration of the drug and its frequency or schedule of administration

Equivalent fraction

Fractions that have the same value

Fahrenheit

System to measure temperature, commonly used in the United States; freezing point of water is 32 °F and the boiling point is 212 °F

Fraction

Numerical representation that indicates a part or a division of some whole

Grain (gr)

Basic unit of weight measure in the apothecary and avoirdupois system

Glossary of Common Terms Related to Pharmacy Calculations

Gram (g)

Unit of weight in the metric system

Heterogeneous

Composed of different substances or different phases [solid/liquid/gas] of the same substance; a mixture where different substances can be clearly seen within the mixture

Homogeneous

Composed of a "uniform composition or structure"; a mixture that appears the same throughout

Household system

Most commonly used system of measuring liquids in outpatient settings

Improper fraction

Numerator is equal to or larger than the denominator; improper fractions are equal to or greater than 1 and can be rewritten as mixed numbers

Intravenous (IV)

Method of medication administration directly into a patient's vein

IV Piggybacks (IVPB)

Composed smaller volumes of fluid "piggybacked" or infused through the fluid of a large volume IV using the same administration set

Liter (L)

Unit of volume in the metric system

Medication order

Prescription in an inpatient or institutional setting

Meter (m)

Unit of length in the metric system

Metric system

Decimal system based on multiples of 10 (0.001, 0.01, 0.1, 1, 10, 100, 1,000, etc.)

Minim (℔ or ℔)

Basic fluid (volume) measure in the apothecary system

Mixed number
Fractions that include both a whole number and a proper fraction

Mixture
Composition of two or more substances that are not chemically combined with each other and are capable of being separated

National Provider Identifier (NPI)
Number issued by the National Plan & Provider Enumeration System (NPPES) to health care facilities and practitioners and often required by third party payers and insurance companies

Numerator
Top number of the fraction; the part

Parenteral
Method of medication administration directly into a patient's vein

Percent (%)
By the hundred or in a hundred

Percentage
Parts per hundred

Prescription
An order to take certain medications, use certain medical devices or a course of treatment

Proper or common fractions
Fractions with a numerator less than the denominator

Proportion
Comparison of two ratios

Ratio
Expresses a relationship between two numbers, usually separated by a colon (:)

Roman numerals
Number system based on Latin letters that are combined for a sum (or difference) of their values

Simplified division

Method of converting a percent to a decimal by shifting the decimal point two places to the left

Simplified multiplication

Method of converting a decimal to a percent by shifting the decimal point two places to the right

Solute

Substance that is dissolved in another substance (a solvent), forming a solution

Solution

Mixture in which particles of one or more substances (the solute) are distributed uniformLy throughout another substance (the solvent), so that the mixture is homogeneous at the molecular or ionic level. The particles in a solution are smaller than those in a suspension

Solvent

Substance that can dissolve another substance, or in which another substance is dissolved, forming a solution

Suspension

Mixture in which small particles of a substance are dispersed throughout a liquid where when left undisturbed, the particles are likely to settle to the bottom; particles in a suspension are larger than those in a solution

Total Parenteral Nutrition (TPN)

Intravenous solutions containing protein, dextrose, electrolytes and/or fat

Volume

How much space a substance occupies

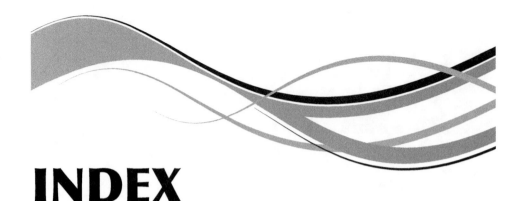

INDEX